Fundamental Fitness After Fifty

Three at Home Fitness Programs to Keep You Functionally Fit For Life

Beth Oldfield

Beth Oldfield can be reached at www.betholdfield.ca

Published by Prominence Publishing www.prominencepublishing.com

ISBN: 978-1-988925-18-9

First Edition: February 2018

AUTHOR'S NOTE

Why write a fitness book? So many have been written already. Bookstores are full of exercise manuals and the internet is ripe with free information. What could I possibly have to offer that would be new and exciting?

The truth is, my fitness students have been asking me to write a book for years. The prospect frightened me but I simply couldn't find a suitable exercise manual on the market today to direct them to, that would cater to their specific needs as active agers. I knew that I had to write one myself! I came to understand that they wanted to be able to do the exercises that we do in class, within the comfort of their own home, on days when they could not make it to the gym. I teach many different levels of fitness so I decided to create a book that could be used by beginner to advanced students alike.

I have helped to keep my students in excellent shape for the last twenty years. Many of them started with me after they themselves turned fifty, so I know that the exercises work and I believe that they are fundamental to healthy living.

I dedicate this book to all of the students who have stood by me over the years. Your faith in me has been uplifting and your strength, determination and dedication has kept me going no matter the weather or the crazy situations that came up during our time together. I have been a witness to your successes and your personal struggles and throughout it all you have taught me so much about life and the resilience of the human spirit. I am so proud of you.

"Reach up, making yourself taller than you were when you walked in."

I say the quote above at the end of every class when we are stretching because I want my students to know that they should be proud for being proactive about their health. Stand tall!

I also dedicate this book to my children Josh, Sarah and Jesse who may want to get into the gym one day. Now at least you can see firsthand what your Mom has been up to all of these years!

With much love,
Beth

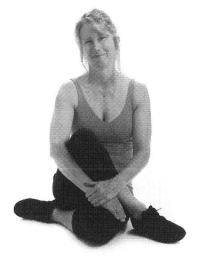

FOREWORD

By Andrea Dewar, B.Sc., P.T

For more than 12 years I have crossed paths with Beth working as a physiotherapist in a sports medicine clinic. Together we have collaborated on many occasions trying to figure out the best approach for injury management and well-being for her clients, my patients and even ourselves.

Never have I met an instructor so dedicated to keeping people of all ages fit. From my end, I hear countless praise for Beth's incredible motivation and uplifting energy during her classes. It is of no surprise the line ups for her classes are literally outside the gym doors.

Beth is an inspirational teacher who cares so deeply about the wellness and health of her students that she dedicates herself to comprehending the finest anatomical details of the human body. This book shows us the key to being stronger, happier and confidant as we embrace the years after 50.

Congratulations to my friend and colleague.

Andrea Dewar – (B.Sc. P.T) Physiotherapist at Action Sport Physio in Montreal since 2001.

WHAT PEOPLE ARE SAYING ABOUT BETH OLDFIELD

"I am 65 years old and I attend on average, 5 hrs of fitness classes a week. Beth's class sets the pace for the week, mentally and physically, for me. Beth's pep and enthusiasm is infectious and so is her smile, always reminding us to "smile" and work every part of our body. I know, at this stage in our lives, our shape won't change much, but we can improve our strength, balance and flexibility. I know I have , and as a bonus, the comradery I feel with all my exercise buddies helps me feel connected and improves overall mental well-being. I love starting my week with "sweat" and "smiles" in Beth's class and a few laughs too. Keep up the good work, Beth. Your fan for almost 18 years."

— Meta

"Staying fit is helping me to be as healthy as possible both in mind and body. This is my job! Now that I am retired I have no excuse but to "get on it" everyday whether it's taking part in Step, aerobics, yoga, stretch, walking, skiing, swimming, biking, gardening. Maintaining a high quality of life for as long as possible is the goal. Experiencing the "joy" is the bi-product."

— Pat, age 68.

"It isn't hard to say how I feel about Beth's fitness classes - I am totally addicted! I feel so lucky to have the opportunity to exercise every day with such a professional and dedicated teacher. Beth's classes are fun and energetic and at the same time, relaxing and calming! I feel that I am challenged to do my best every day but am always reminded "to listen to my body" and not to push beyond my capabilities that day. My daughter just challenged me to do a side plank on an extended arm, and I was able to do it! I am sure I could not have done that four years ago when I first retired from teaching and joined the 3F program. I am now 62 years old and feeling more fit than ever! Thanks so much for guiding us all towards fitness for life in such a positive way!"

— Judy

"It was about 14 years ago when I was 50 that I reluctantly pushed myself to a fitness class to give it a try, feeling it was time I started doing something extra to help my body cope with the inevitable aging process. I did not find it an easy class but Beth happened to be the teacher and it was her enthusiasm and encouragement that kept me going. At first it was a struggle but Beth and the group just became part of my routine. Beth gets to know us all, making the class more personal, telling us stories during Plank, helping us through various injuries and she notices when we are missing so I became very dedicated and rarely missed a class. I have attended many of Beth's classes over the past 14 years, and though I am retired now, with life and grandchildren at times getting in the way, I still try very hard not to miss class. My body and I thank you Beth for continuing to encourage and inspire us, making us believe you can keep us going well into our 90s!!"

— Sandy

viii   Fundamental Fitness After Fifty

"Like many other people, I have physical challenges to face. When the arthritis took hold (I now just call it "my friend Arthur") it took away many things. My fatigue was overwhelming. My joints were painful. And sometimes I could barely make it home from work. But I took Beth's early morning class anyway. She always said to do what I could – but also made it clear that she expected me to do at least that much! The camaraderie she fosters, her enthusiasm, and her range of exercise programs, her encouragement... all this so important to learning to enjoy physical activity again.

"And Beth got me into the habit of exercising, even when it was almost too painful. There was always a benefit, and there were many more good days than bad, thanks to the exercises. You made my life bigger and my disease smaller. Thank you!"

— Margaret

"37 years in and still going to the gym and pool. 14 of which were with Beth who never gave up on the over 50s. Thanks to regular exercise and good food I'm able to keep fit and healthy not forgetting the company of good friends."

— 73 year old Step student

"After 35 years of classes I feel I have kept fit in both mind and body. Arthritic knees have made me change some classes but "stretching" has always been a favourite for sure. Another plus are the good friends I have made over the years."

— Joan Swail, age 75

"I've been doing fitness classes for the last 33 years. I am now 82 and certainly know this has kept me going –especially the last 15 years, when age was becoming a factor. Beth's step class was excellent-then my arthritic knee kicked in and so I changed to Aqua-fitness. I once was told by my Osteopath that the best thing at this age is to "stretch," So...have been doing Beth's Yoga stretch for 2 years now and it certainly has been great on the joints. Beth seems to have a keen understanding of what seniors need in exercise. To keep moving is so important to the body and mind as well. Good luck Beth-have enjoyed your "blog" so much and your classes."

— Audrey

"I have been taking classes with Beth for over 10 years. In 2015 I retired from working at age 63. I immediately signed up for fitness classes at Beth's main place of work. At first I was doing 2 step classes a week besides walking on average 200 kilometers per month. I then added the ball class to the step classes while continuing the walking on a daily basis. Almost one year later, I am much stronger in most muscle groups and graduated from using 5 and 7 pound weights to 8 and 10 pound weights. Also, my stamina is much better for walking long distances. I am able to do things I could not do a year ago such as get up off the floor without getting on my hands and knees and superman swim on the floor.   I am not motivated to work out on my own so having Beth's classes available is very important to me and I hope she never retires!"

— Paul.

"I was one of those people who joined fitness clubs. It always turned out to be money wasted because I would stop going. Everything else seemed more important until I got older and started breaking bones.

Several over a period of five years. Unknowingly, I had osteoporosis and paid greatly for my sedentary life. I had to get serious about working out and started attending Beth Oldfield's classes. That was four years ago, and the benefits are many. Not only am I physically stronger, but I have also incorporated Beth's many suggestions into my daily life. I breathe better, watch my posture, work on my balance, and even sit and get out of chairs more carefully. I also walk more and keep active. I may break another bone someday, who knows? But if I do, I will be better equipped to achieve full recovery."

— Diane

"I was never a person who liked to exercise on a mat on the floor and I never could touch my toes (still can't). Flexible didn't describe me. When I retired, I knew I needed to keep moving and a friend recommended Beth's class. After one session, I was hooked. Beth has a vibrant personality and strives to know each student by name. I enjoy the weight training, balance and stretching exercises that are part of the program. I also started to learn line dancing from Beth and have challenged my body and mind while dancing to the great music. I feel young again when I'm dancing! Through these courses, I have improved my balance, body tone and have lost weight. My bone density test results have improved (while also being augmented with medication). I look forward to being in your classes for many more years!"

— Linda Haynes

"I have known my trainer, Beth Oldfield, since 2003. What I like about Beth is how diverse her competencies are and her concern for the well-being of her students. She comes up with new routines monthly. She offers appropriate exercises that challenge her students no matter their fitness level. I wish I had met her earlier in my life. Thank you for keeping me in good shape."

— Mariette

"I suffered two broken legs after a car accident. I had a year of physio after the accident, then joined some fitness classes. For the next year or so I felt my legs were getting stronger and less painful all the time but then I seemed to plateau and I began to think that maybe this is as good as it gets. Then Beth started the line dancing class and everything changed! I didn't know if I would be able to do it at first, I thought I would be falling over my feet, but I could do it! And it was so much fun and I was so thrilled I was almost in tears. However, that night I was in pain from my hips to my toes, but it soon got better, so I kept going back to class and each time the pain was less, until now I have no pain as such. There has been enormous improvement in my movement since I started dancing. I always felt it was more than just the exercise. It was as if the free movement (as opposed to controlled exercises) re-awakened pathways between my brain and the nerves and muscles in my legs. So I can't thank you enough, Beth! Not just for this and my specific case, but for all of us who benefit from your excellent classes and your caring encouragement and inspiration – and yes, your smile too!"

— Diana

"I am forever grateful to have been in Beth's classes last year. When I arrived for my first day, Beth asked me what I was looking for in this course. I explained that I had back problems and wished to make it stronger. Because Beth made my back stronger, I was able to go through several months of really hard physical work to renovate my property following the spring floods in 2017. I couldn't have crawled into the very confined space under my house to take away and install new insulation. Not one contractor wanted to do this job that is how difficult it was. I was also able to redo my patio with 2' x 2' cement tiles, and transport and install a big concrete fence! I enjoyed Beth's professionalism, competency, and her diversified training programs and her nice personality. Now that my renovations are almost done, I'll be back!"

— Lucie

"I'm happy to have Beth as a trainer and to be part of her fitness classes. I feel all the physical benefits as well as the psychological ones. She takes such good care of my whole being. I only have one wish: to have Beth in my life for a very long time. Thank you Beth for keeping me in good shape. To our friendship, Carole"

— Carole

"I have been training with Beth for five years. When I started taking her classes, I had just come out of a major depression and addiction to alcohol and drugs. My sister Carole encouraged me to join Beth's fitness group and the exercises gave me energy, self-confidence and stability. I once again found the will to live a clean, healthy life. Because of Beth, I am strong and fit!"

— Ginette

TABLE OF CONTENTS

INTRODUCTION

Thank you for purchasing *Fundamental Fitness After Fifty.* I look forward to helping you on your journey toward improved health.

I am a personal trainer and fitness instructor with twenty years of experience in the fitness field. I've been specializing in training people aged fifty and older for more than 15 years. I know what exercises work because my students have remained healthy despite any physical setbacks brought on by injury or disease. I currently train clients in their mid-fifties to mid-eighties and I am inspired daily by their success!

I will not be tackling diet in this book but I want you to understand that we really are what we eat! You cannot expect your body to perform at its best if you are fueling it with empty calories. I recommend eating a balanced diet that includes many vegetables and varying protein sources.

When it comes to losing weight and what will work best for you, I always tell my students to seek the advice of a nutritionist. One way to start is to write down everything that you eat and drink for a week. Be honest and you will see where you might be able to lose weight simply by changing the foods that you are consuming. And don't forget to put alcohol consumption on your list. It is amazing how readily those innocuous glasses of wine or liquor add up to unwanted weight gain. Speak to your doctor before making any drastic changes to your eating patterns and medications.

How to Use This Book

Section I breaks down the fundamental exercises that you need to do in order to remain functionally fit for life. I want you to be able to do the activities that you love, long into your later years and you should be successful if you devote some time each day to your health.

Section II is divided up by exercise intensity. You will find exercises with detailed instructions for Beginner; Intermediate and Advanced. To complete the work in each section, students will need a small playground ball, a set of weights and a mat. All of these are readily available at any store that carries fitness equipment.

Beginning students will be using a chair so please chose one that is sturdy with a backrest. Feel free to begin in the Beginner section and progress through to the harder levels as you gain strength and confidence.

Section III details the stretches that you need to do at the end of each workout. I use the chair for the stretches because it is suitable and effective for all levels of fitness. These stretches can be done daily if you choose after an initial warm up of your muscles.

Safety First

I tell my students that, "if something hurts, STOP."

Remember that you must listen to your body and if any movement causes you pain, stop immediately and seek the advice of a health care professional. It's normal to feel stiffness after exercise and be aware that you can feel fine and then experience pain or stiffness two days later.

It is important to warm up before you begin the exercises. You can achieve this by walking for five to ten minutes. Move your arms back and forth as you walk to generate heat in the shoulders.

Ideally the exercises in this book are completed two to three days per week, with one days rest in between the workouts. In other words, give your body a day off from training so that your muscles can recover and grow. If you do these workouts on back to back days you risk injury. Do the exercises in the order listed.

Try to pick a weight that leaves you feeling tired by the last repetition. You do not want the exercises to be so easy that you do not feel as though you have worked at all. That being said, you want to be able to complete the set amount of repetitions.

In most cases you will be doing 15 repetitions of each exercise. If you feel tired by 12 repetitions that is fine. You will build up strength over time. Some of the exercises will have you holding the pose for 20-30 seconds. Be careful to read the instructions carefully.

"Tip from your hip," or hip hinge forward whenever we are in a forward folding position. You can place your fingers where your body naturally bends at the top of your hip to remind yourself to keep a straight back when bending forward. Do not round your lower back during these exercises unless you are stretching.

Stretch after the workout by following the last section of the book and hydrate properly during and after the session.

I hope that my book will help you to reach your fitness goals and enjoy a long, pain free and active life!

Let's begin.

SECTION I

WHY THESE EXERCISES?

I believe that the most important exercises to do regularly are the ones that keep us functionally fit. If we think about the movements that we do often and the muscles that are used in those actions, we want to focus on keeping the muscles involved strong and flexible.

Many of my clients love to participate in activities such as golfing, curling, hiking, biking and gardening. All of these require strength; flexibility and balance. Even though you may have been actively participating in these sports for the last twenty years, the only way to guarantee that you will enjoy another twenty pain free, is to formally train the muscles involved.

The hard truth is that we can still get injured despite being in good physical health. I have had several injuries that my physiotherapist has remedied and because of these experiences, I value fluidity of movement above everything else. I want to remain flexible; strong and independent long into my golden years and I want the same for you!

We also heal much faster when we are good physical condition.

Fundamental Movements

The human body is designed to **Push**; **Pull**; **Lift; Bend**; **Squat**; **Lunge** and **Twist**.

When you think about the flow of your day all of these movements are necessary. We have to train all of the muscles involved in these motions for strength and flexibility and not just the ones that we use in our favorite activities. The body needs to be well balanced because when it is not, injuries can occur from doing simple movements.

For example, we can feel quite healthy one moment and then twist to turn and pick up something and strain our back. Often we are left wondering what happened when really the imbalance has been worsening over time unbeknownst to us. This is why I always suggest attending different fitness classes; changing your training program every six to eight weeks and participating in a variety of physical activities so that we do not build up these imbalances in the first place.

Let's imagine the flow of your day and the muscles that you need to move freely.

We take it completely for granted but getting out of bed requires abdominal and arm strength. I know this because I slipped a disc in my back years ago and simply rolling over in bed was almost impossible. Any of you who have suffered back pain know how many muscles we need to recruit to rise up from our beds in a pain free manner.

Showering requires twisting and bending as we move about the shower stall reaching for products. Picking up the soap that fell to the floor or washing our feet, requires not only balance and stability but flexibility. Getting in and out of the bathtub requires strength in our arms, legs and core.

Putting on our socks, and pants requires forward bending as well as balance and coordination. Most of us sit to put these items on but we should be able to stand and perform these tasks and if not, we still need the flexibility in our spine to bend forward from a sitting position. Getting on our bras, shirts and tank tops requires healthy, flexible shoulders and dexterity. I can remember getting into a tiny changing room once with a pull over blouse that was probably a bit too small for me. Well, I got it on but could not easily get it off and believe me I was very grateful that my shoulder flexibility was there that day or I may still be stuck in that teeny room with the blouse half over my head. I panicked that day and have never aimed to fit into that size again!

Grocery shopping often requires reaching for products on top shelves or lifting heavy boxes (think bulk stores). Even if someone assists us in getting the products out of the store and into our car, we still need to be able to lift them out of the trunk and or the backseat and into our home. Add the challenge of a heavy snowfall to this mix or freezing rain and watch the difficulty level increase.

Cooking often requires getting equipment that may be high up in the cupboards or squatting down to get into lower cabinets. My mixer is very heavy and bulky and to get it out, I have to be able to squat down and lift it to the counter. If we don't have the luxury of a mixer, kneading bread dough by hand requires a tremendous amount of wrist strength and beating batters requires shoulder endurance.

Driving requires flexibility in the neck to check blind spots and we need to be able to get in and out of the car seat. When I slipped my disc in my back, all of this was very painful, not to mention pushing on the gas pedal. I once had an injured shoulder and shifting gears was hard to do pain free, as was simply lifting a kettle full of water.

While I can't promise that you will never get injured if you exercise, I know from personal experience that we heal better and quicker if we are in good physical shape. When we do get injured, our physio's have us start recovering by addressing the weakness that caused the situation to unfold. We heal by going back to the basics of simple movement and building up our strength where it is needed.

I design all of my programs keeping these fundamental movements in mind. My mission is to keep my students strong and flexible so that daily tasks are easy and activities can be fully enjoyed.

Abdominal Exercises

You will see that I have picked non-traditional abdominal exercises for my book because we are very familiar with typical sit-ups where we lie on our backs, hands at our head and curl our shoulders upward. Please feel free to do these but remember not to pull on your head and to keep a space between your chin and chest.

Instead of sit-ups, you will find V-sit exercises on both the chair and on the mat. The focus is on lengthening your torso, instead of crunching toward your knees.

In both cases, it is important for you to recognize any back pain or neck pain. While it is normal to feel a tremble in your abdominals during the movement, pain should be avoided. If you prefer traditional abdominal work, replace the V-sits however you see fit, but I do advise that you seek the services of a qualified trainer for guidance to address your concerns specifically.

Posture is Key

Stand up please and have a look at yourself in a full length mirror.

I want you to roll your shoulders up and then back and down. Move your chin back instead of pushing it outward. Now imagine that there is a string pulling you upward from the top of your head. Lengthen through your abdominals, depressing your shoulders slightly. Chances are that you look as though you have just lost a pound or two.

We spend so much time hunched forward in both our work and free time (think watching television or sitting on the couch on our electronic devices) that we have a hard time actually sitting and standing tall. If you exercise in bad posture, you will get injured. In all of the following exercises, be certain to check your posture first by doing the movements exactly as described.

The Importance of Stretching

When I first started teaching twenty years ago, the industry did not encourage us to spend more than five minutes stretching at the end of a fitness class. I began to notice that my students were in need of more and so I began to devote at least ten minutes at the end of every class to rebalance the body after our workouts. In 2011, I began to teach hour long stretch classes.

Please remember that you have to make the time to stretch out your muscles after your workout to prevent injuries. I am currently learning to teach Essentrics, a full body stretching and strengthening program because I see how important it is for us to be long and lean and strong.

Remember to follow the stretches at the end of this program. I also recommend joining a gentle yoga class or find an Essentrics class in your area. Never push to the point of pain and if something hurts, speak to a healthcare professional.

SECTION II

THE EXERCISES

The Beginner Workout

You are at a beginner training level if you have not attended fitness classes before or worked with a personal trainer. While you may be physically active some of the time, you are not familiar with fitness equipment, the gym environment and common exercises. If you have suffered a knee or back injury and you want to be extra cautious, I recommend that you start with this section of the book. You want to build up your strength, balance and flexibility without putting too much pressure on your joints.

You will be using a chair in order to take the load off of your knees and to help with posture and balance. Remember to start with light weights but you can increase the weight as you gain strength. You want to be able to complete the repetitions but it should not be too easy or too hard.

Before beginning these exercises, spend ten minutes enjoying some form of cardio such as walking and then do the following exercises in the order listed. Unless otherwise stated, do 12- 15 repetitions of each exercise.

For your convenience all of the photos of the exercises are laid out on two pages at the end of this section to make it easier to follow along. Once you know how to execute the exercises properly, this feature will allow you to work more quickly.

Remember to stretch after you are done by following the stretches listed in Section III.

1. Ball Wall Squat

A. Begin: Stand with your back to the wall with the little ball behind your back. Feet are hip distance apart and out from the wall.

B. Active: Lower down until your knees are bent at 90'. Your knees should be stacked directly over your ankles. If you experience knee pain, simply lower to a pain free range of motion. Keep your back straight with your head lined up over your tailbone. Return to the starting position. Repeat 12-15 times.

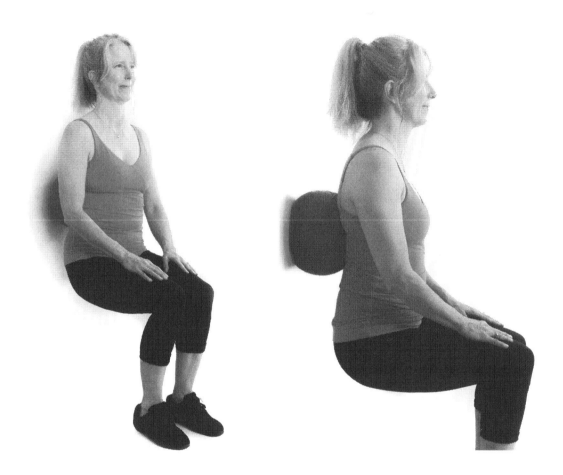

2. Wall Push-up

A. Begin: Place your hands wide apart on a wall surface, while standing a few feet away.

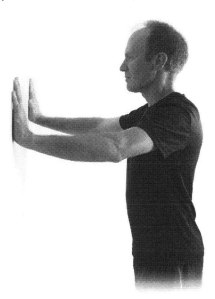

B. Active: Lower your chest toward the wall, keeping your back straight. You may prefer to come onto your toes. From the lowered position, look toward your elbow, it should line up with your shoulders. Your hands should be lined up under your elbow which is bent at 90'. Push back up to the starting position. Repeat 12-15 times.

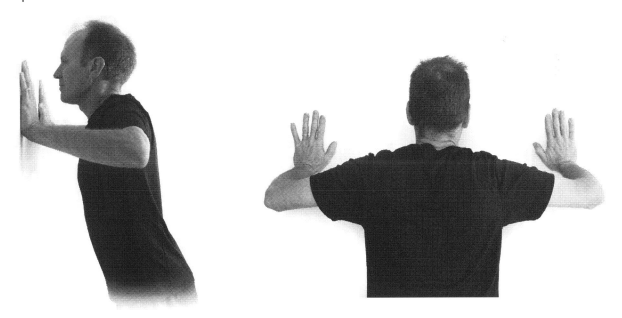

3. Front Arm Raise

A. Begin: Sit tall on the front edge of the chair with weights in your hands, arms hanging down by your side, with palms facing in.

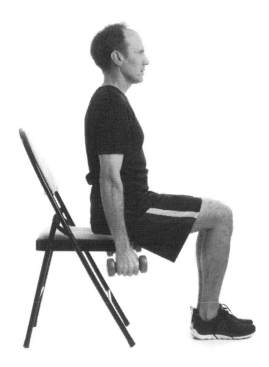

B. Active: Raise your arms up in front until they are in line with your shoulders. Your thumbs should be facing up. Lower back down to the starting position. Repeat 12-15 times.

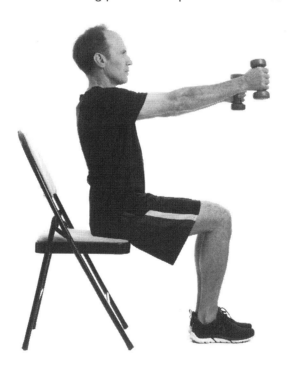

4. Split Squat

A. Begin: Stand to the right side of your chair with your right foot forward and your left hand on the backrest of the chair. Your left leg is extended to the back, behind your left hip and you are on the toes of the left foot.

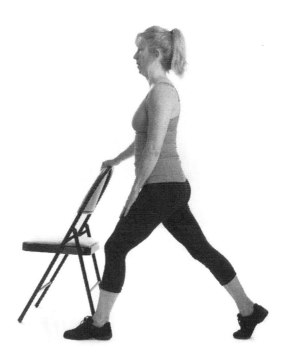

B. Active: Lower down until your right knee is bent at 90' or to a pain free range of motion. Rise back up again and repeat all reps on this side and then do the reverse on the other side. Complete 12-15 repetitions.

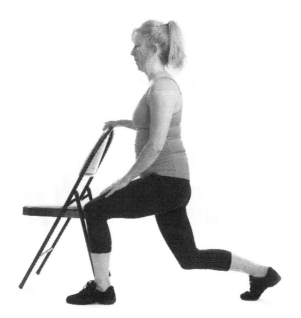

5. Bicep Curls

A. Begin: Sit tall on the front edge of your chair with weights in your hands, arms hanging down by your sides, palms facing forward.

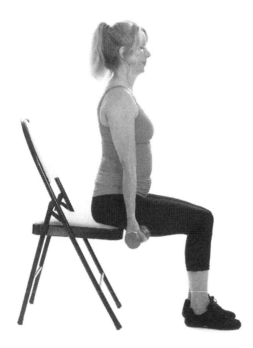

B. Active: Keep elbows by your sides as you curl your hands toward your shoulders. Don't lift your hands all the way up to the shoulder. If you feel your elbows leaving your side you have lifted too high. Lower back down to the beginning position. Repeat 12-15 times.

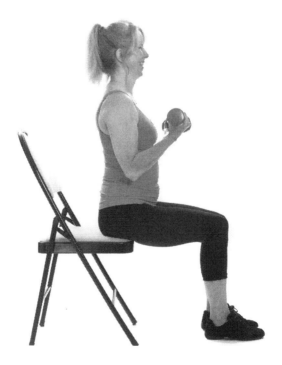

6. Standing Superman

A. Begin: Stand to the right side of your chair. Place your left hand on the backrest of the chair and extend your left leg to the back, in line with your hip and rest onto the toes.

B. Active: Tip forward from your hip until your upper body is parallel to the floor and raise your left leg up until it is even with your hip while extending your right arm out in front. Keep your back straight. Keep your head in line with your spine and your right arm should remain in line with your right ear. Return to the start position. Repeat 12-15 times and then complete this exercise on the other side of the chair with the opposite arm and leg.

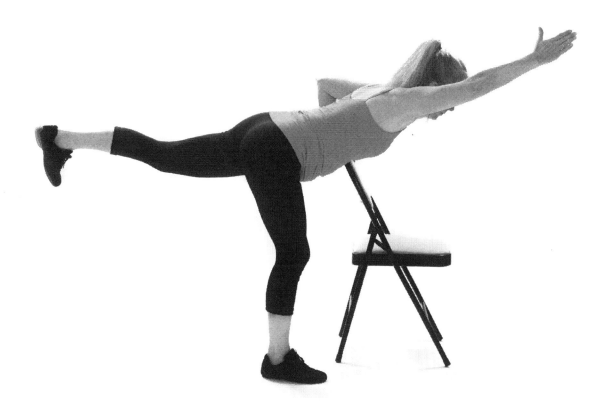

7. Abdominal Exercise – Push and Resist

A. Sit tall on the front edge of the chair, lift your right knee just a bit while pushing down on it with the right hand. Do not let your knee be pushed down. You should feel your abdominals tighten up. Release and repeat with the other knee and hand.

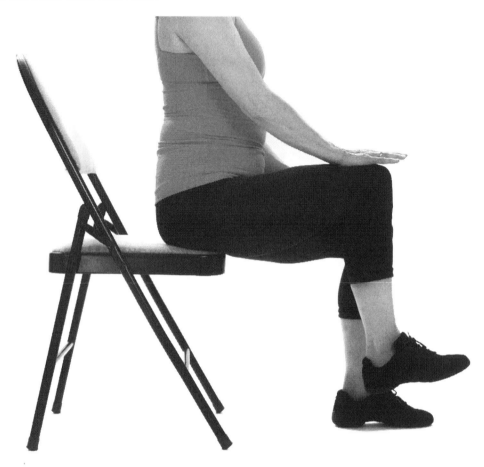

8. Bent Row

A. Begin: Sit tall on the front edge of the chair with a weight in your right hand, arm extended toward the ground, palm facing in. Hip hinge forward and rest your left arm across your knees to support your upper body.

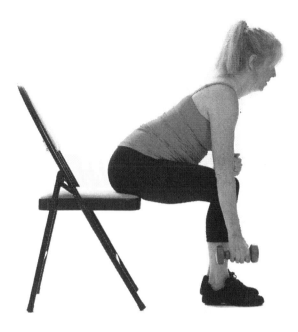

B. Active: Pull your elbow up to pass your back, while keeping your shoulders even. Do not twist your body by raising your right shoulder. Lower back to the start position and repeat all reps, then do the left arm. Complete 12-15 repetitions.

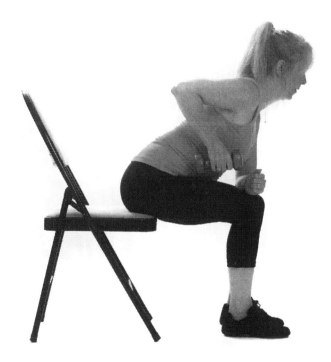

9. Abdominal Exercise with the Ball

A. Begin: Sit with the ball placed on the chair behind you, braced against the back of the chair, sit with your lower back against the ball, with your hands at your head. Easier option is to have hands crossed over your chest.

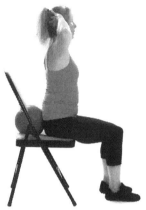

B. Active: Contract your abs as you lower backwards without touching your shoulders to the chair and hold. You should feel your abdominals shake a bit. Keep breathing and then return to the starting position. Complete the reps.

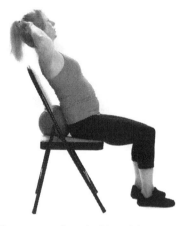

C. Progression: Start the exercise with arms extended beside your ears.

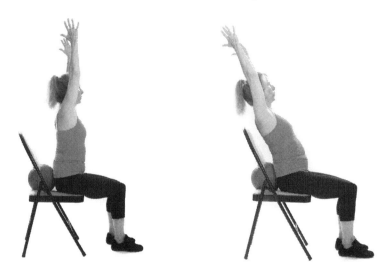

10. Triceps Extension:

A. Begin: Sit tall on the front edge of the chair with a weight in your right hand, palm facing in. Hip hinge forward and rest your left elbow across your knees to support your upper body. Pull the elbow up passed your back. Wrist in lined up under the elbow which is bent at 90'. This is the starting position.

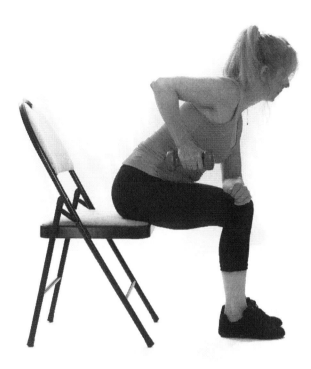

B. Active: Straighten your right arm behind you and then return to the 90'bent position. Repeat 12- 15 times and then do the same with the left arm.

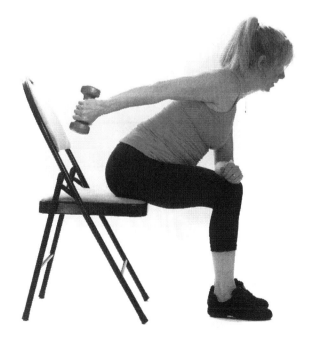

11. Abdominal (Oblique) Work with the Ball

A. Begin: With the ball placed on the chair behind you, braced against the back of the chair, sit with your lower back against the ball, hands at your head. Easier option is to have the hands crossed over your chest.

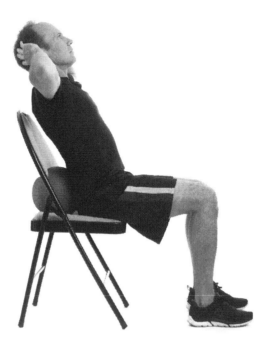

B. Active: Contract your abdominals and lean backwards without touching your shoulders to the chair and hold. Now slowly rotate your shoulders to the left and then to the right. Return to center and then rise back up. Remember to breathe throughout the exercise. Repeat 12-15 times.

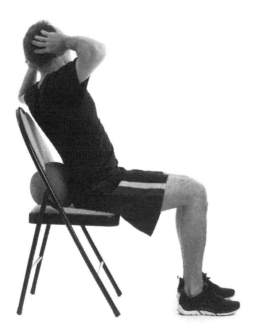

C. Progression: Have your arms up in the air beside your ears. Not pictured.

12. Lateral Arm Raise

A. Begin: Sit tall on the front edge of the chair with weights in your hands, arms hanging down by your side, with palms facing in.

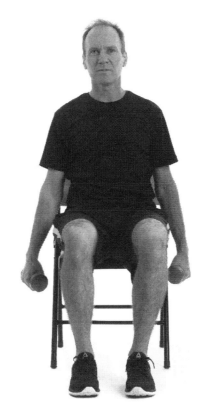

B. Active: Raise arms up out to the side until they are even with your shoulders. Lower back down to the starting position. Repeat 12-15 times.

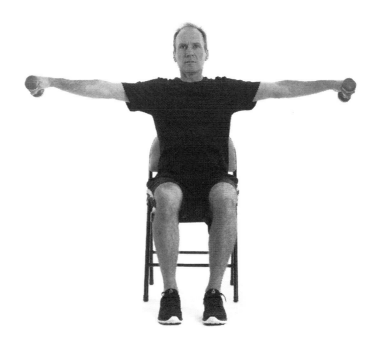

13. Balance

A. Begin: Stand to the right side of the chair and rest your left hand on the backrest of the chair. Raise your left knee. Contract the muscles of the supporting leg and your abs.

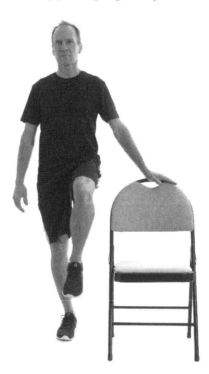

B. Active: Try to lift your hand off of the chair. Hold for a count of 5. Repeat 8 times and then try the other side.

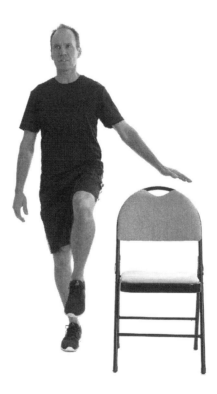

14. Balance with Rotation:

A. Begin: Stand to the right side of your chair with your left hand on the backrest of the chair. Raise your left knee. Contract the muscles of the supporting leg and your abs.

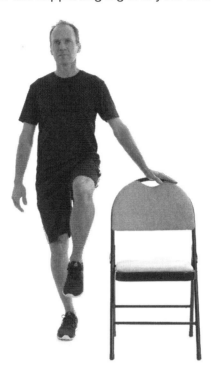

B. Active: Turn your upper body toward the chair and now try to lift your hand off of the chair. Hold for a count of 5. Repeat 8 times and then try the other side.

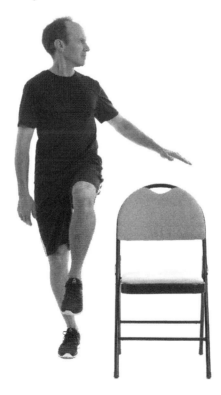

Quick Glance Summary

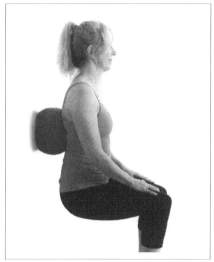

1. Ball Wall Squat

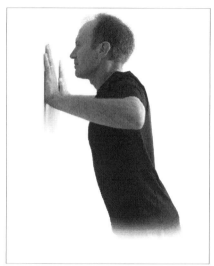

2. Wall Push-Up

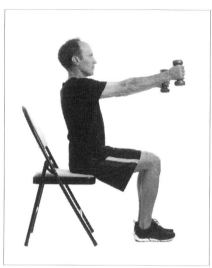

3. Front Arm Raise

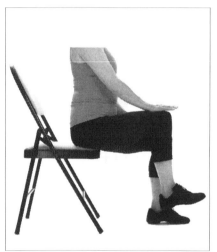

7. Abdominal Exercise – Push and Resist

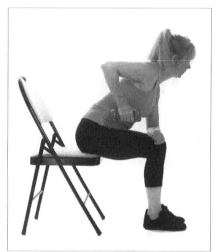

8. Bent Row

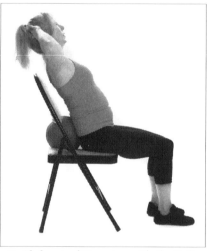

9. Abdominal Exercise with the Ball

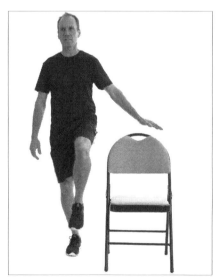

13. Balance

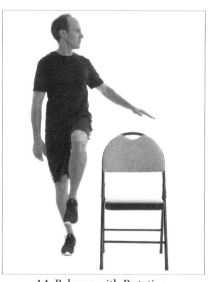

14. Balance with Rotation

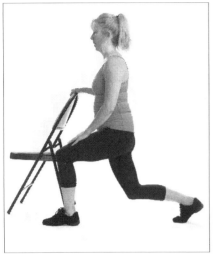

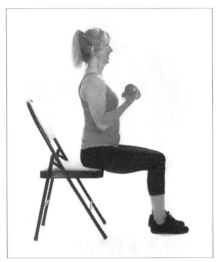

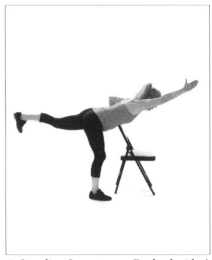

4. Split Squat – Do both sides!　　　5. Bicep Curls　　　6. Standing Superman – Do both sides!

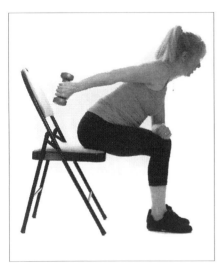

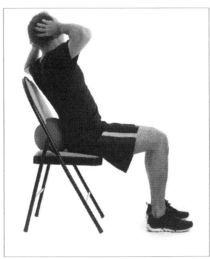

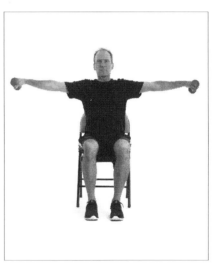

10. Triceps Extension　　　11. Abdominal Exercise (Oblique)　　　12. Lateral Arm Raise
with the Ball

The Intermediate Workout

You are at an intermediate training level if you attend fitness classes at least two times per week or have worked with a personal trainer on a regular basis. You are familiar with basic exercises and you like to be challenged. You enjoy a level of flexibility that allows you to get down onto an exercise mat. Though your joints may be stiff, you are very active and want to improve your strength and balance.

As you gain strength you can chose to go through the program twice, effectively completing two sets of each exercise. I recommend doing the whole program from start to finish before beginning a second set. Remember to select a weight for lifting that allows you to complete the repetitions. It should not feel too hard or too easy, so adjust accordingly.

Before beginning these exercises, spend ten minutes enjoying some form of cardio such as walking and then do the following exercises in the order listed. Unless otherwise stated, do 12- 15 repetitions of each exercise. In some cases you will be holding a pose for 20-30 seconds. In this case, you only do the movement only once.

For your convenience all of the photos of the exercises are laid out on two pages at the end of this section to make it easier to follow along. Once you know how to execute the exercises properly this feature will allow you to work more quickly.

Remember to stretch after you are done by following the stretches listed in Section III.

1. Front Raise:

A. Begin: Stand tall with weights in your hands, with your palms facing inward toward your thighs.

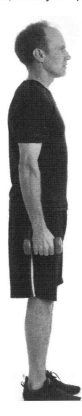

B. Active: Raise your arms to shoulder height, with your thumbs pointing up as if you were hitch hiking. Lower back to the starting position and repeat 12-15 times.

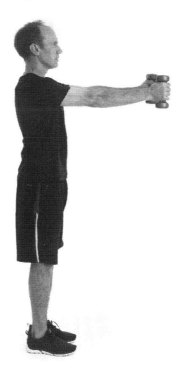

2. Squat:

A. Begin: Stand tall with feet under your hips, hands by your side.

B. Active: Bend your knees as you tip forward from your hip, keeping your back straight. Send your hips to the back and arms out in front to help with balance. Lower down until your knees are bent at 90' or slightly above.

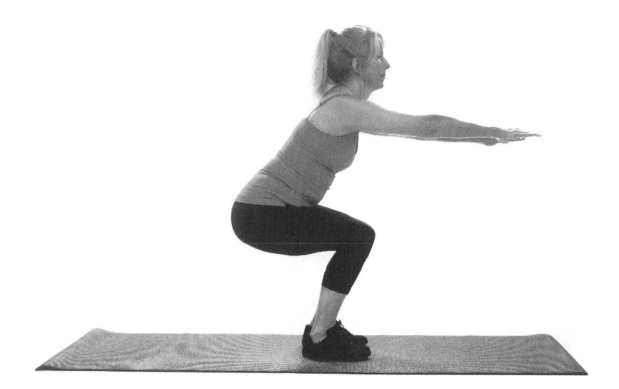

3. Overhead press:

A. Begin: Stand tall with weights in your hands. Place your arms up in the air, elbows out to the side and bent at 90' with your palms facing outward.

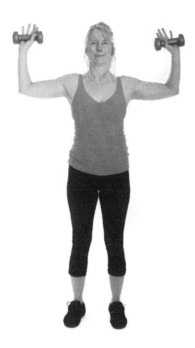

B. Active: Raise your arms up overhead and lower back down to the starting position. Keep your back straight. Do not push your hips forward and sink into your lower back. Stay tall!

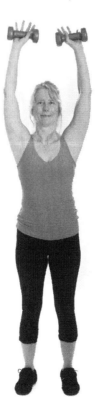

4. Split Squat:

A. Begin: Stand tall with weights in your hands, palms facing inward. Note: picture is missing the weights. Extend your right leg backward onto the toes.

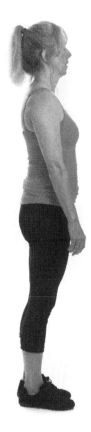

B. Active: Lower down until your knee is bent at 90' or slightly higher. Rise back up keeping the leg behind you and then lower down again to complete 12-15 repetitions

Then perform the exercise with left leg behind.

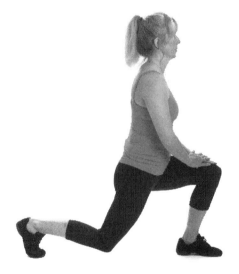

5. Bicep Curls:

A. Begin: Stand tall with weights in your hands, palms facing outward.

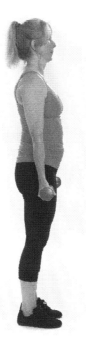

B. Active: Lift the weights toward your shoulders, keeping your elbows by your sides. If you feel your elbows start to come forward, you are lifting too high. Lower back down and repeat to complete 12-15 repetitions.

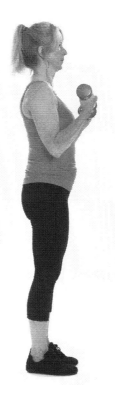

6. Push Ups:

A. Begin: Come down onto your hands and knees onto the mat. Move your knees slightly backward behind your hips and have your hands wide apart, probably off the sides of the mat. An easier option is to have your knees directly under your hips.

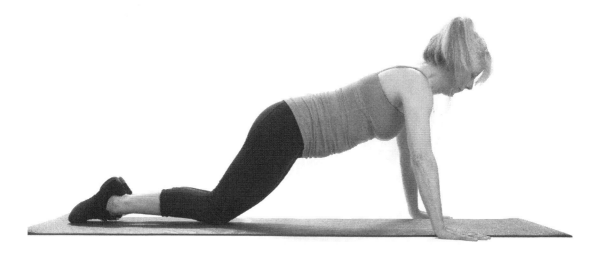

B. Active: Lower your chest toward the floor until your elbows are bent at 90'. Keep your elbows lined up over your wrists. Your chest should be between your hands, not your face. Imagine that there is a string lined at your fingertips and put your nose over that imaginary line.

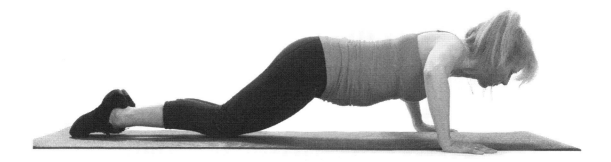

7. Prone Straight Arm Raise:

A. Begin: Lie face down on the mat, with your arms down by your hips, palms facing upward with a weight in each hand.

B. Active: Keep your head down as you lift your arms upward. Lower down and repeat. If you want it to be harder, do not lower completely to the floor after each lift but stay slightly above the mat.

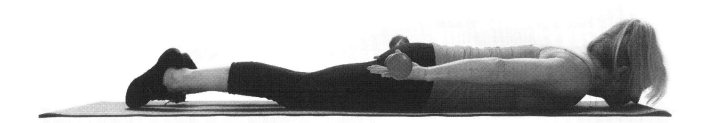

8. Plank:

A. Begin: Lie on your belly with your hands and forearms on the mat.

B. Active: Contract your abdominals and lift your pelvis and stomach off of the mat, coming onto your elbows and knees which are behind your hips. HOLD for 20-30 seconds. Remember to breathe throughout. Progression is to build up to 1 minute.

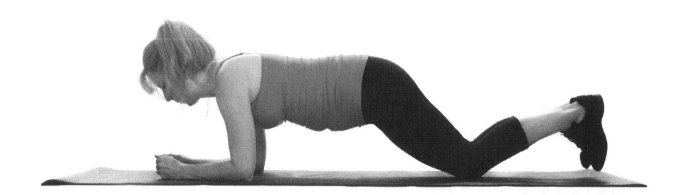

9. Superman:

A. Begin: Lie on your stomach with your arms out in front of you on the floor.

B. Active: Raise your right leg and left arm at the same time and then lower down, repeating with the left leg and right arm. This completes one repetition. Repeat 12-15 repetitions.

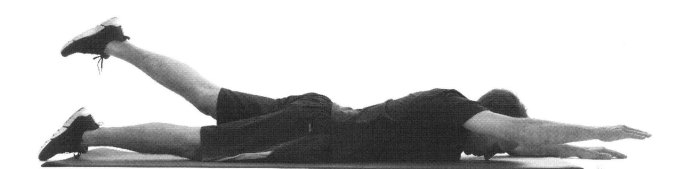

10. Side Plank: Knees or Feet:

A. Begin: Prop yourself up onto your elbow while lying on your side. Elbow is lined up under the shoulder. Knees are bent and slightly forward.

B. Active: Lift your hips off of the mat coming onto your knees with your top arm reaching upward in line with your shoulder. Keep your head in line with your spine. HOLD for 10-20 seconds. Repeat on the other side.

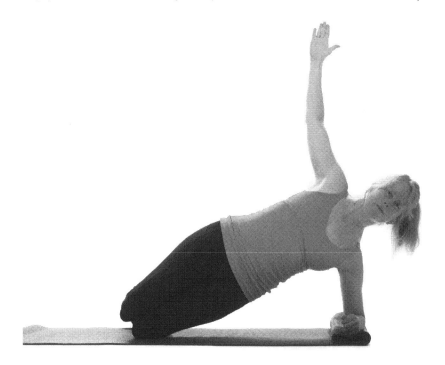

C. Progression: Lift your hips off of the mat coming onto your stacked feet, with the legs straight.

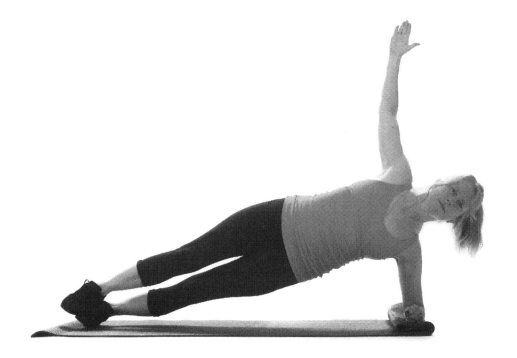

11. Skull Crushers:

A. Begin: Lie on your back with weights in your hands, near the top of your head, palms facing inward. Keep your elbows in, do not let them fall out to the sides.

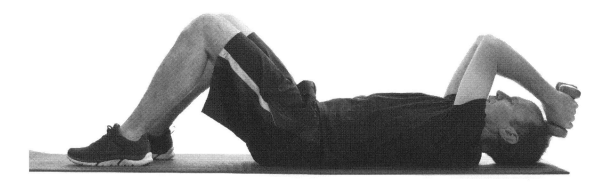

B. Active: Without moving your elbows forward, straighten your arms upward toward the ceiling. Return to the starting position and repeat 12-15 times.

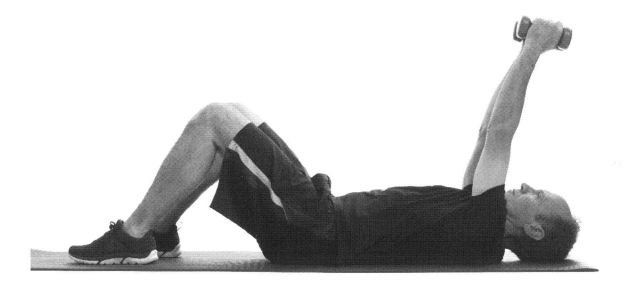

12. V-Sits with the Ball:

A. Begin: Sit tall on the matt with knees bent and feet on the floor. Prop the ball behind your lower back so that it will not move. You will have to lean back on it slightly to keep it still.

B. Active: Cross your arms over your chest, contract your abdominals and then lower backward, until you feel your abdominals start to shake. Hold for 3 seconds and rise back up. Repeat 10 times.

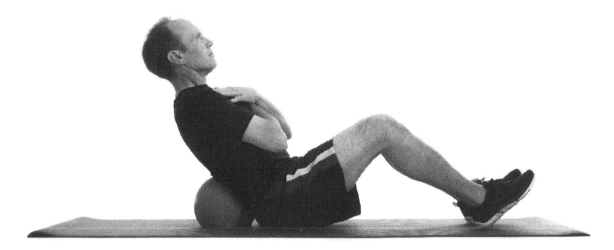

C. Progression: Have your hands at your head.

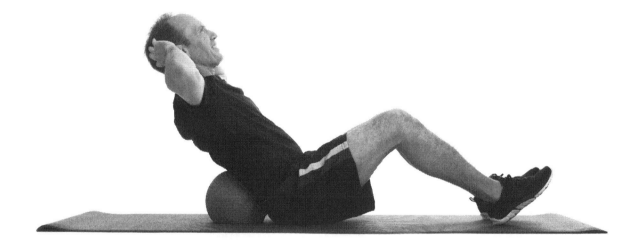

13. Balance:

A. Begin: Stand tall and hold the ball in your hands, resting it on one knee that is raised up in line with the hip. Keep the muscles of the supporting leg contracted along with your abdominals and buttocks

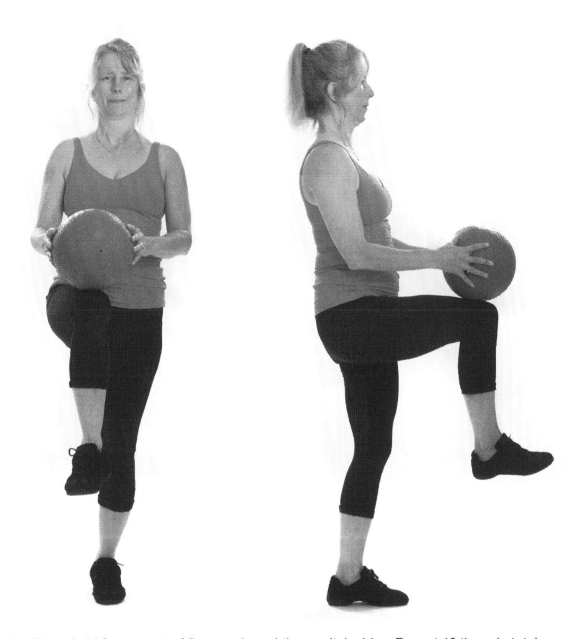

B. Active: Try to hold for a count of 6 seconds and then switch sides. Repeat 10 times in total.

14. Balance with Rotation:

A. Begin: Stand tall with the ball in your hands, one knee raised in line with the hip. Keep the muscles of the supporting leg contracted along with the abdominals and buttocks.

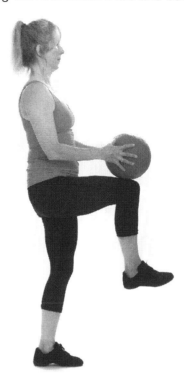

B. Active: Turn your body and arms toward the knee, bringing the ball to the outside of the knee. Hold momentarily and return. Do 10 rotations and then switch sides.

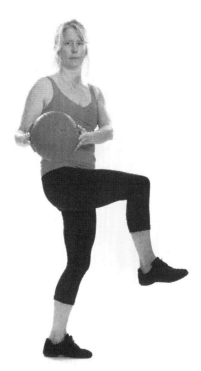

Turn the page to see a recap of all the Intermediate exercises on one page.

Quick Glance Summary

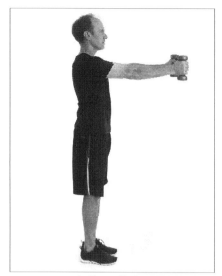

1. Front Raise

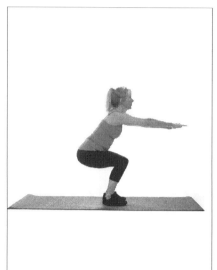

2. Squat

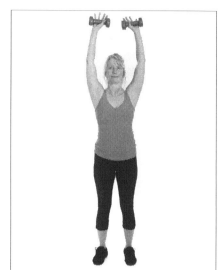

3. Overhead Press

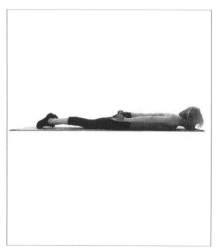

7. Prone Straight Arm Raise

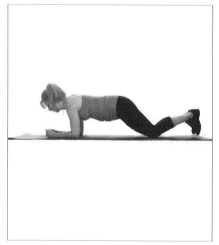

8. Plank

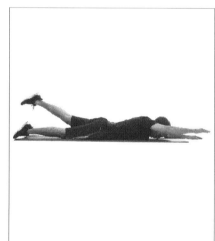

9. Superman – Opposite Arm and Leg

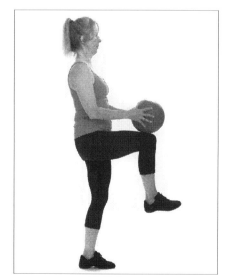

13. Balance

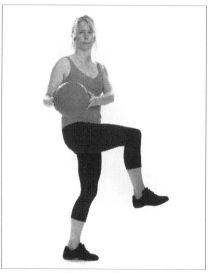

14. Balance with Rotation

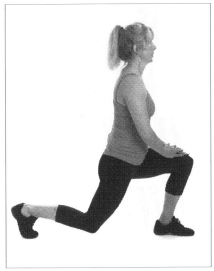

4. Split Squat – Do both legs

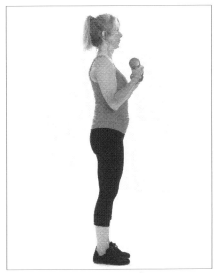

5. Bicep Curl

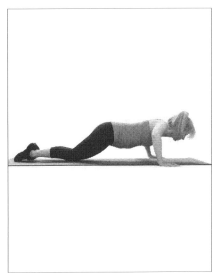

6. Push-Ups

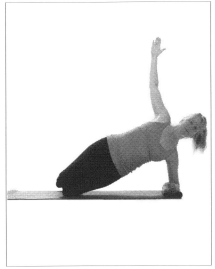

10. Side Plank – Knees or Feet

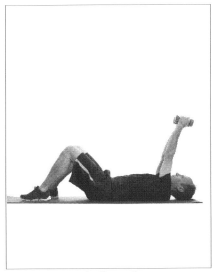

11. Skull Crushers

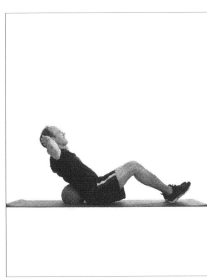

12. V-Sit with the Ball

The Advanced Workout

You are at an Advanced training level if you have been attending fitness classes three or more times per week for an extended period of time or you have been weight training under the supervision of a personal trainer regularly. You enjoy a pain free, active lifestyle and love to be challenged physically with interesting exercises that improve strength and balance.

Before beginning these exercises, spend ten minutes enjoying some form of cardio such as walking and then do the following exercises in the order listed. Unless otherwise stated, do 12- 15 repetitions of each exercise. Remember to select a weight that challenges you. It should not be too hard or too easy so adjust accordingly. In some cases you will be holding a pose for 20-30 seconds. In this case you only perform the exercise once.

As you gain strength you can chose to go through the program twice, effectively completing two sets of each exercise. I recommend doing the whole program from start to finish before beginning a second set.

For your convenience all of the photos of the exercises are laid out on two pages at the end of this section to make it easier to follow along. Once you know how to execute the exercises properly this feature will allow you to work more quickly.

Remember to stretch after you are done by following the stretches listed in Section III.

1. Back Lunge with Knee lift holding weights:

A. Begin: Stand tall with weights in your hands, palms facing inward with right knee raised.

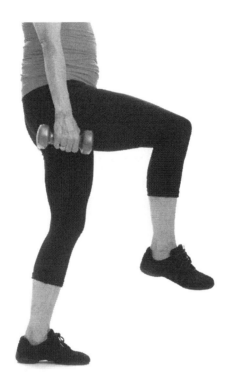

B. Active: Take a big step backward with the right leg, coming onto the toes. Using your left leg, lift up the right leg and bring your right knee up in front. Try not to push off with your right toes. Really use the left leg by pushing down through your heel to rise back up. Repeat all reps and then switch to the other leg.

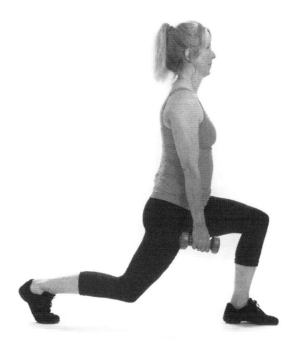

2. Bicep Curl: One Arm/Standing on One Leg

A. Begin: Stand on right leg, with left knee up in line with left hip and both weights in your right hand, palm facing front.

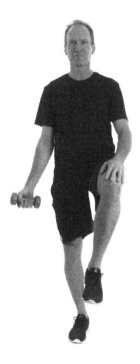

B. Active: Curl your hand toward your shoulder but keep your elbow by your side. When you feel your elbow start to come away from your side, you have lifted high enough. Lower back to the starting position and repeat. Complete 12-15 repetitions and then switch to the other leg and arm.

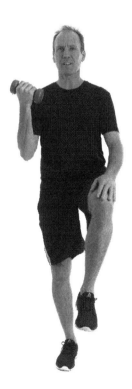

3. Walking Squat:

A. Begin: Get down on your right knee on the mat with your left foot on the floor in front. Left knee is bent at 90'. Right knee under your hips.

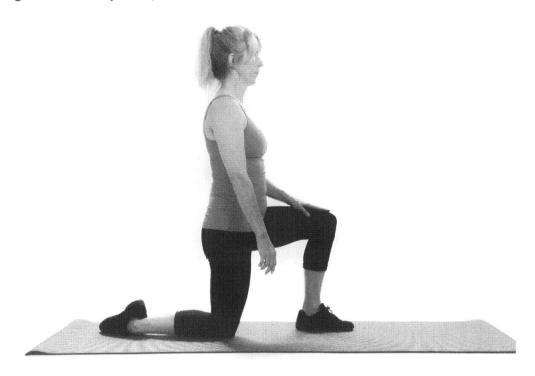

B. Active: Raise your right knee and put your foot on the floor in front of you coming directly into a squat, hold and then replace your right knee to the mat and then your left. Begin again by leading with the right leg. Keep alternating sides for a total of 12 to 16 repetitions.

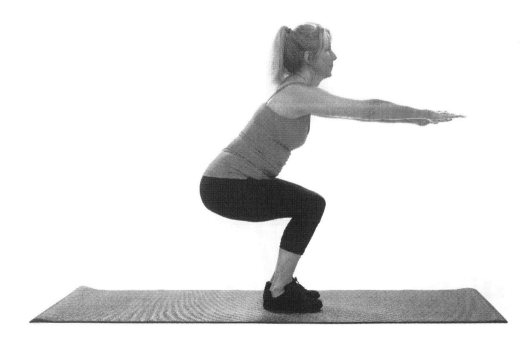

4. Overhead Press: One Arm Standing on One Leg:

A. Begin: Stand on your right leg with the weight in your right hand, left knee lifted in line with the left hip and your right elbow bent at 90'. Palm facing outward.

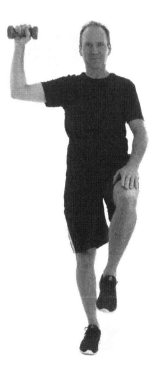

B. Active: Straighten your right arm up toward the ceiling and then lower it back down to 90' at the elbow. Keep the left knee lifted at all times. Complete 12-15 reps and then reverse so that you are standing on your left leg, right knee in line with your right hip and the weights in your left hand.

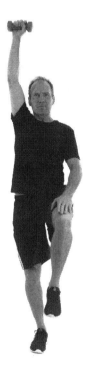

5. Dead Lift:

A. Begin: Stand tall with weights in your hands in front of your thighs, palms facing inward.

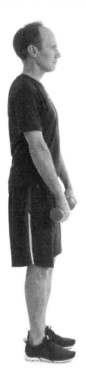

B. Active: Send your hips backward as if coming into a squat while you keep your back straight. Your arms will hang down straight and your hands will dip below your knees. Rise back up again, using your legs to get back up. To do this contract the muscles in the back of the legs (hamstrings) to return to the starting position. Keep your head in line with your spine.

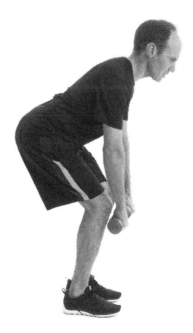

6. Plank with Leg Lifts:

A. Begin: Lie on your stomach on the mat. Prop yourself up onto your forearms and toes. Make sure that your elbows are under your shoulders and that your back is flat. Imagine that you are like a straight plank of wood.

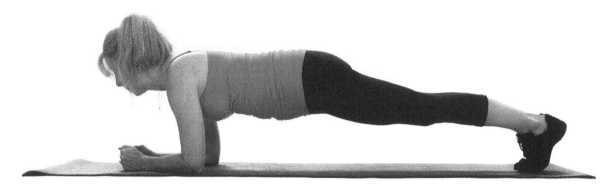

B. Active: Lift a toe and hold for 3 seconds and then switch sides. Maintain a straight back. Do 10 repetitions.

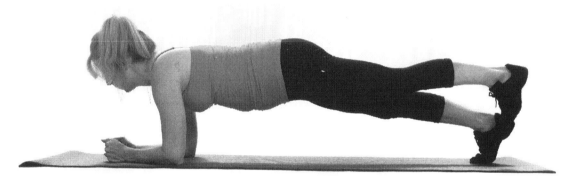

7. Triceps Push Ups:

A. Begin: On your hands and knees on the mat, with knees behind hips and hands under your shoulders.

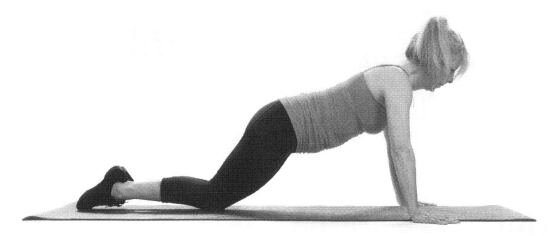

B. Active: Lower your chest toward the floor, keeping your elbows by your sides. Imagine that you are going to lie your ribs onto your bent arms. Rise up and repeat 12-15 times.

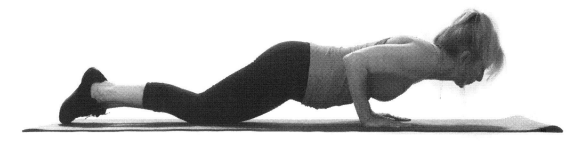

C. Progression: Do the above exercise from your toes.

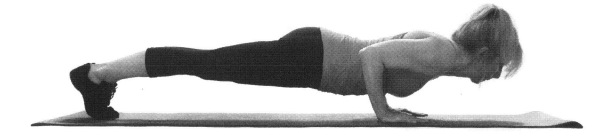

8. Quad Box Row:

A. Begin: On your hands and knees, with knees under the hips and hands under the shoulders, hold both weights in your right hand and extend your left leg behind the hip and rest it on the toe.

B. Active: Raise your right arm and left leg, bending the arm to bring the elbow up past your back and raising the leg to be even with the buttocks. Complete 12-15 reps with the right arm and left leg and then switch to the other side.

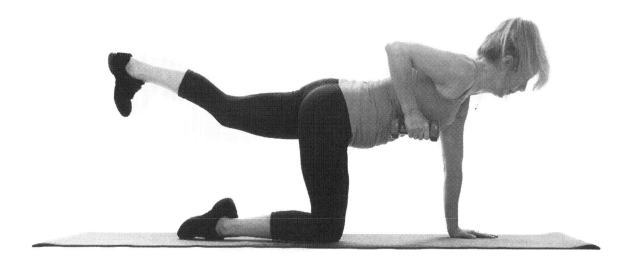

9. Side Plank with Rotation:

A. Begin: Lie on your side. Prop up onto your forearm and your stacked feet with your top arm extended upward, in line with your shoulder.

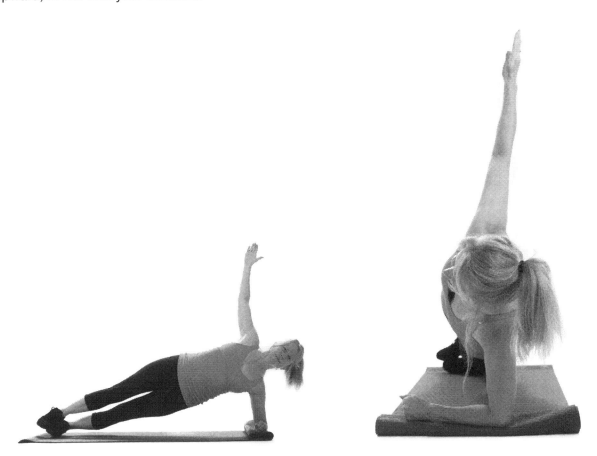

B. Active: Bring the extended arm downward, turning your shoulders toward the mat as if you were going to turn to the other side but don't. Straighten yourself back up. Repeat 4 rotations and then hold straight up for 10 seconds.

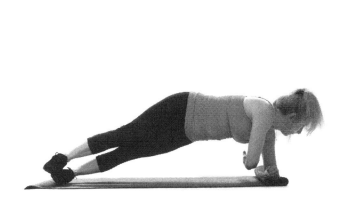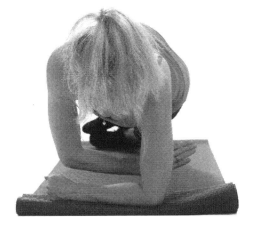

10. V-sits with Ball:

A. Begin: Sit tall on the matt and prop the ball behind your lower back so that it will not move. You will have to lean back on it a bit to keep it still. Your back should be straight. Bend your knees with your heels on the floor. Arms raised up beside your ears.

B. Active: Contract your abdominals and lower backwards, keeping your back straight, until you feel your abdominals start to shake. Hold for 3 seconds and rise back up. Repeat 10 times. You can make this more difficult by holding a lightweight in your hands.

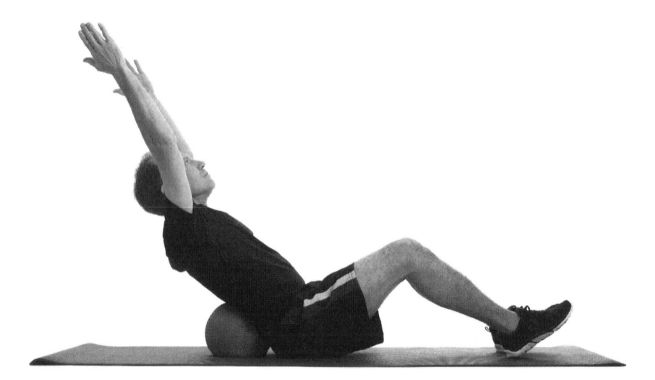

11. Push Ups:

A. A. Begin: Come onto your toes and hands which are placed wide apart, off the sides of the mat.

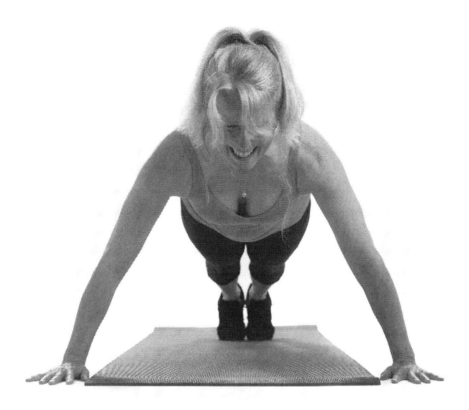

B. Active: Lower your chest toward the floor until your elbows are bent at 90'. Keep your elbows lined up over your wrists. Your chest should be between your hands, not your face.

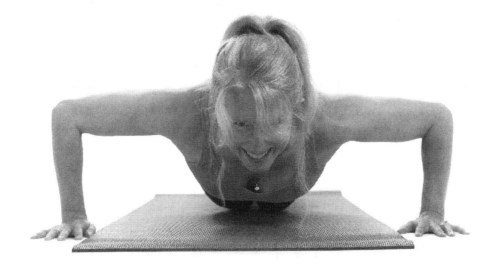

12. Superman:

A. Begin: Lie on the mat on your stomach, with your arms out in front like Superman.

B. Active: Raise both arms and legs at the same time, keeping your head in line with your spine and your chest down on the mat.

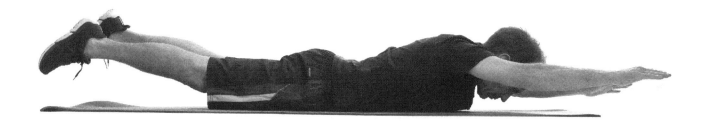

13. Balance with the Ball:

A. Begin: Stand tall with the ball in your hands, right knee raised in line with the hip. Keep the muscles of the supporting leg contracted along with the abdominals and buttocks.

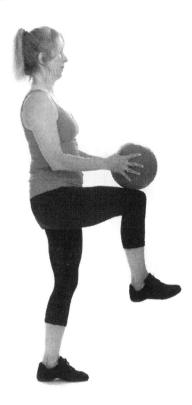

B. Active: Rotate the upper body toward the knee.

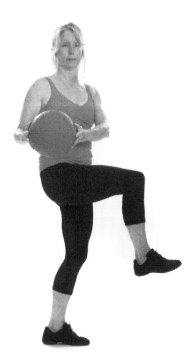

C. Active: Return to face front and then extend the right leg to the back as you tip forward from your hip and extend arms out in front. Try not to touch the right foot down to the floor between repetitions. Keep your hips even and your head in line with your spine as you try to raise your arms up beside your ears. Return to standing tall, trying not to touch the right foot down. Complete 12-15 reps and then switch legs.

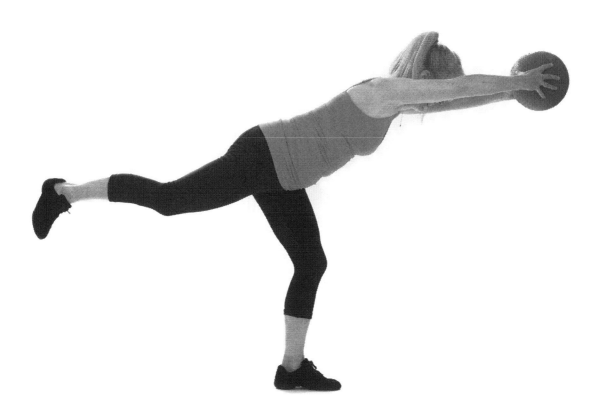

Turn the page to see a recap of all the Advanced exercises on one page.

Quick Glance Summary

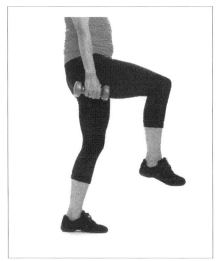

1. Back lunge knee lift with weights

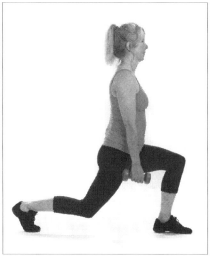

1. Back lunge knee lift with weights

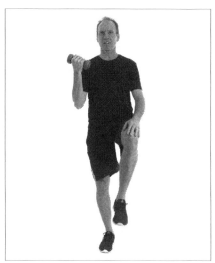

2. Bicep Curl- Do both sides

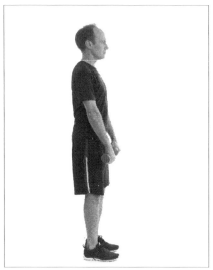

5. Dead Lift

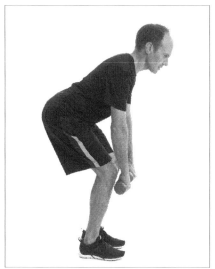

5. Dead Lift

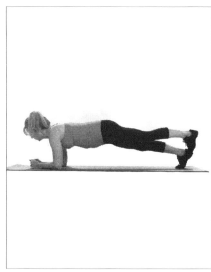

6. Plank – Switch leg lifts 10 times

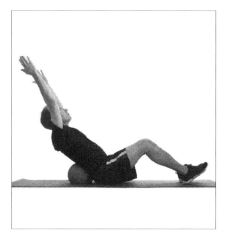

10. V-Sits with Ball – Optional weight in hands

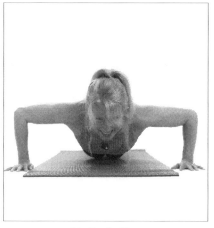

11. Push-Ups

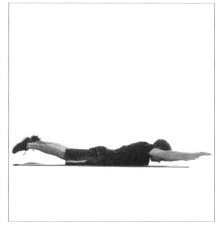

12. Superman

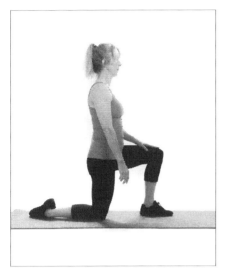

3. Walking Squat

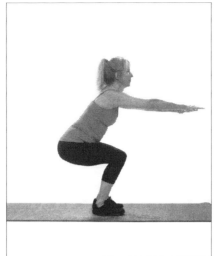

3. Walking Squat

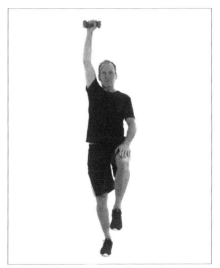

4. Overhead Press – Do both sides

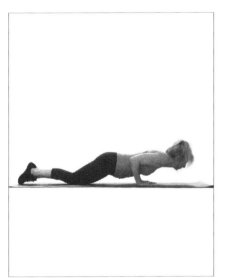

7. Triceps Push-ups – Knees or Toes

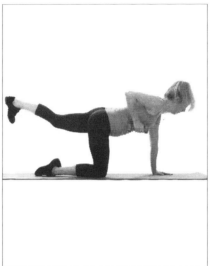

8. Quad Box Row – Do both arms

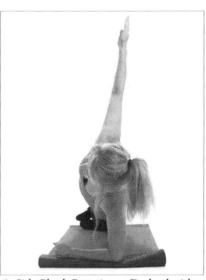

9. Side Plank Rotation – Do both sides

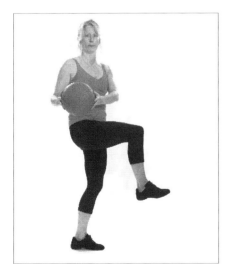

13. Balance – Do both sides

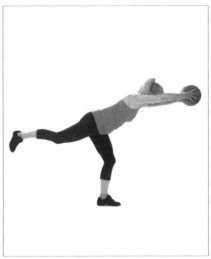

13. Balance – Do both sides

SECTION III

THE STRETCHES

Ease into the stretch until you feel your muscles. Hold the stretch for 3-6 seconds and then try to move into the stretch a little bit deeper and hold for an additional 10-20 seconds longer. You should not experience any pain. Stop if something hurts. Remember to breathe throughout. You can do these stretches daily after an adequate warm up.

1. Open Arms - Chest and Shoulder:

A. Active: Sit tall on the edge of your chair and open your arms wide. Expand your chest.

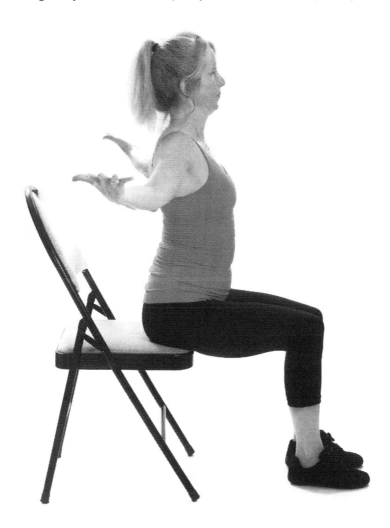

2. Cat Stretch - Back and Forearms:

A. Begin: Sit tall on the edge of the chair and interlace your fingers, and straighten arms with palms facing outward.

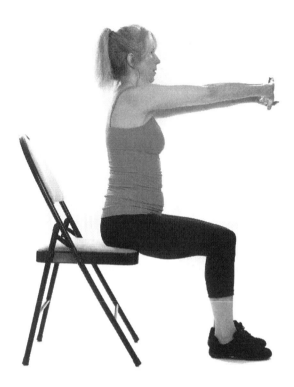

B. Active: Round your back and push your hands toward the front of the room.

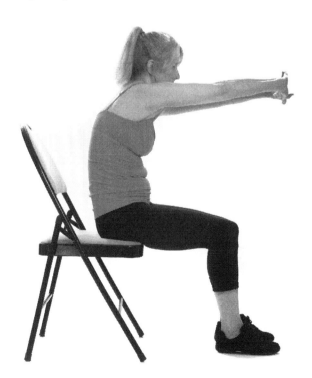

3. Sky Reach - Abdominal (Rectus Abdominis)/Chest/Latissimus Dorsi:

A. Active: Sit tall on the edge of the chair. Raise arms up overhead, reaching for the sky. Lean backward slightly.

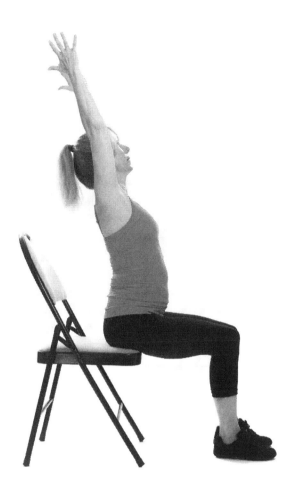

4. Belly Bliss - Abdominal (Rectus Abdominis)/ Chest/ Shoulders:

A. Sit tall on the edge of the chair. Place fists on your hip bones and lean backward so as to open your chest.

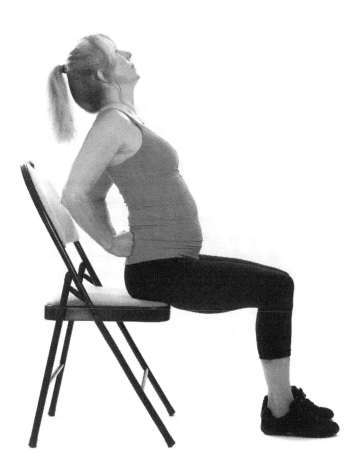

5. Side Opener - Oblique /Latissimus Dorsi:

A. Active: Sit tall on the chair and stretch one arm upward, then lean over slightly. Repeat other side.

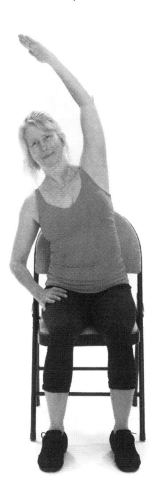

6. Back Scratch – Triceps/Shoulder/Chest:

A. Sit tall with your back against the chair. Raise one arms upward and then place your fingertips on your back. Use the other arm to pull the elbow backward slightly. Lean into the chair to help to keep your back straight. Keep looking straight ahead. Don't drop your chin.

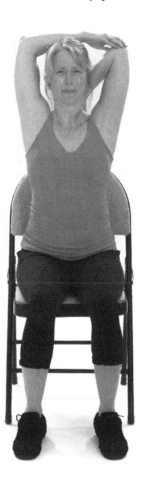

7. One Arm Hug – Upper Back/Shoulder:

A. Active: Sit tall in the chair and bring one arm across your chest, gently pushing it inward with the other hand.

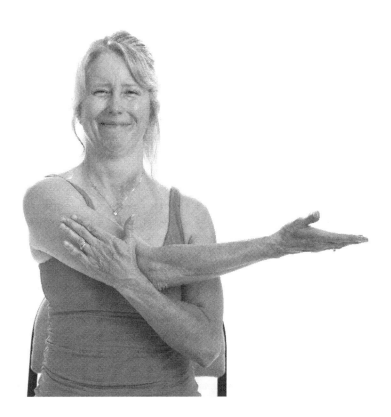

8. Spine Twist - Lower Back/Chest/Shoulder/ Neck:

A. Active: Sit tall on the edge of the chair. Turn your body to the left by first turning your lower back, then your ribs, then your shoulders and finally your neck. Place your right hand on the outside of your left knee, keeping your knees facing front and open up your left arm. Return slowly to the front by turning your neck, then ribs then lower back. Repeat to the other side.

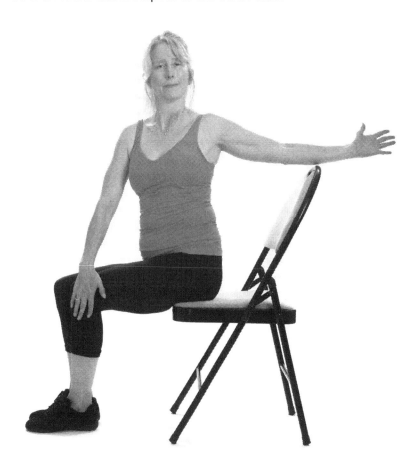

9. Two Arm Hug – Upper Back/Shoulders

A. Sit tall on the edge of the chair and wrap both arms around your shoulders, rounding your upper back slightly.

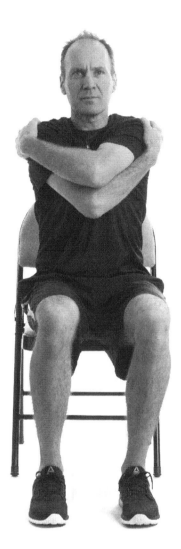

10. Figure 4 – Hip/Inner Thigh/Lower Back

A. While sitting on the edge of your chair, raise one leg up crossing the ankle over the knee. Tip forward from your hip, gently pressing downward on the knee. Repeat with other leg.

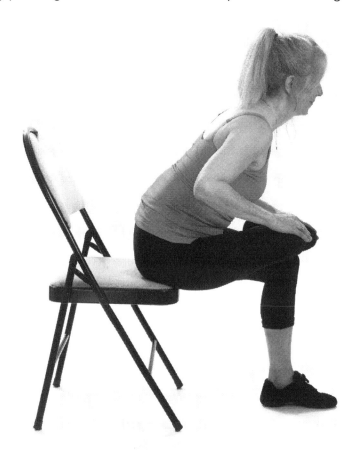

11. Lengthening Lunge - Quadriceps/Hip/Abdominals/Chest/Arms:

A. Active: Sit sideways on the chair and extend your back leg behind you onto the toes while reaching your arms upward. Repeat with the other leg.

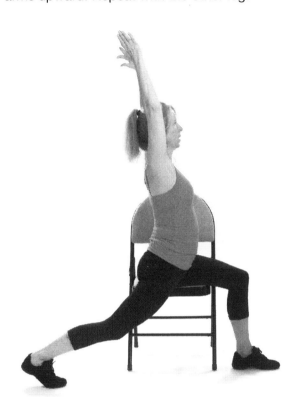
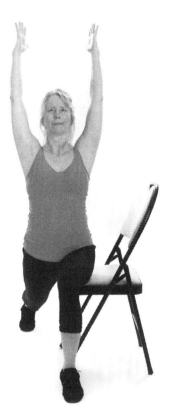

12. Ankle Grab – Quadriceps/Hip/Shoulder:

A. Active: Sit sideways on the chair and grab your ankle, sock or shoe depending on your flexibility level and keep your knee aligned under your hip. Repeat on the other side.

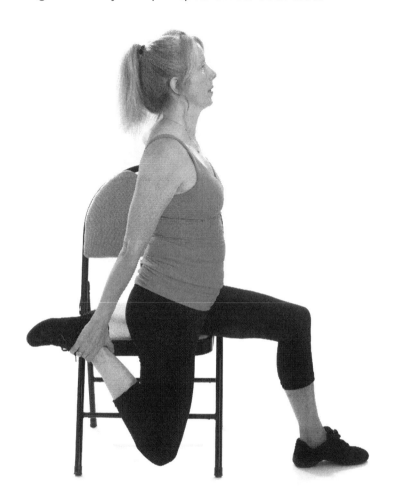

13. Single Leg Toe Reach – Hamstrings/Calf/Lower Back:

A. Active: Sit tall on the edge of the chair and extend one leg it out in front onto the heel. Lift your toes and tip from your hip until you feel a good stretch up the back of your leg.

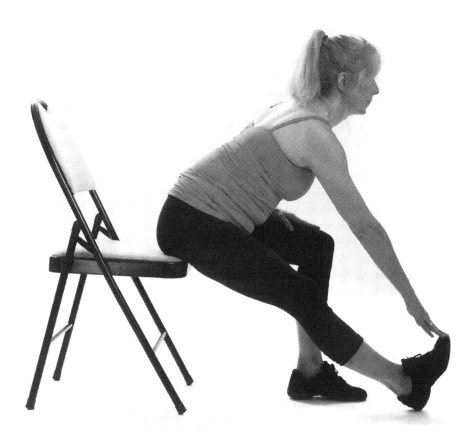

14. Double Leg Toe Reach – Hamstrings/Calves/Lower Back/Arms:

A. Active: Sit tall on the edge of your chair with both of your legs extended out in front onto the heels. Tip from your hip, reaching for your toes until you feel the stretch.

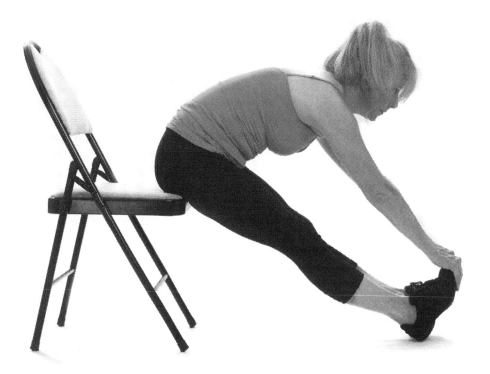

15. Wrist Bliss – Wrist Flexors and Extensors:

A. Active: Extend your arm out in front of your body with your hand facing away from you as if you are telling someone to "STOP" and gently pull your fingers toward you.

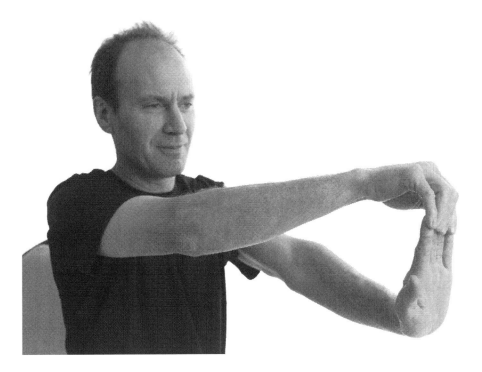

B. Active: With your arm out in front of your body, point your fingers down toward the ground and pull your fingers inward.

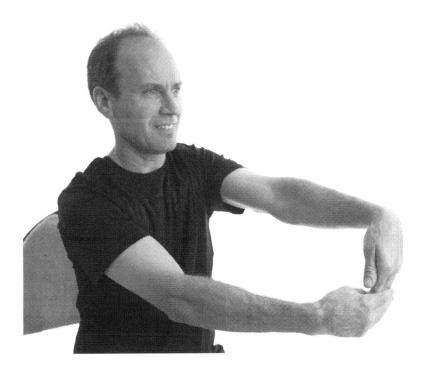

Quick Glance Summary

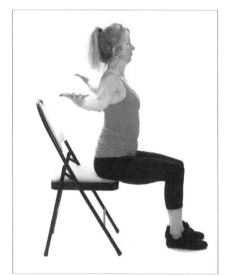

1. Open Arms

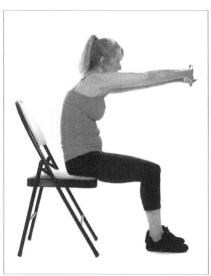

2. Cat Stretch

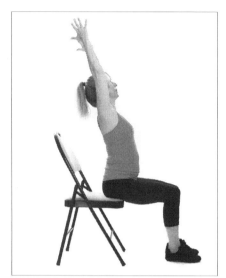

3. Sky Reach

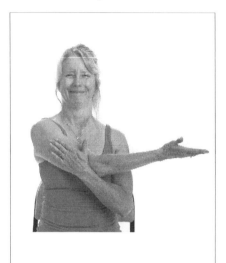

7. One Arm Hug – Do both sides

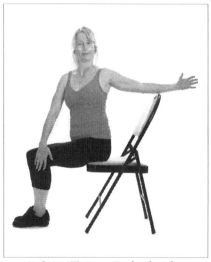

8. Spine Twist – Do both sides

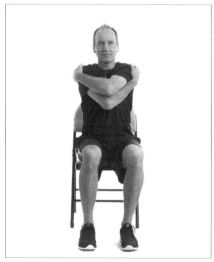

9. Two Arm Hug

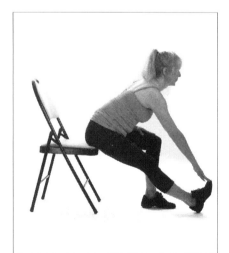

13. Single Leg Toe Reach – Do both sides

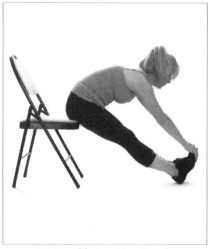

14. Double Leg Toe Reach

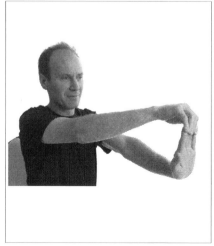

15. Wrist Bliss – Do both arms

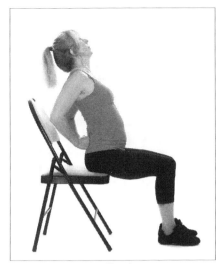

4. Belly Bliss

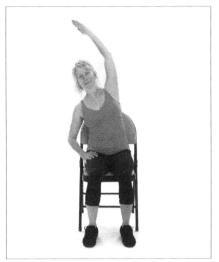

5. Side Opener – Do both sides

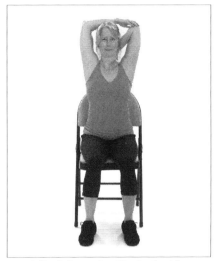

6. Back Scratch – Do both sides

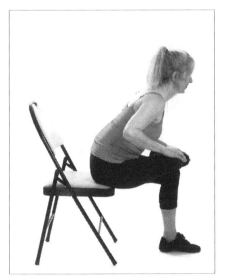

10. Figure 4 – Do both sides

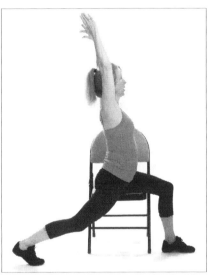

11. Lengthening Lunge – Do both sides

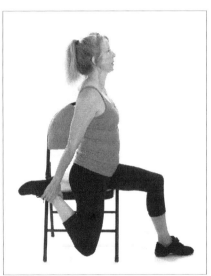

12. Ankle Grab – Do both sides

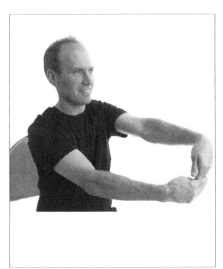

15. Wrist Bliss – Do both arms

TWENTY YEARS OF STORIES

"Don't Tell Me to Give Up Cola!"

When I first met Linda, she was over fifty and really motivated to lose some pounds. I presented her with the fitness program that she would be doing three times per week and then asked her to tell me a bit about her daily diet. Well, the first thing she did was get right up close to my face, wag her finger and tell me that she drinks 6 big glasses cola every day and that she refuses to give that up! I backed off and told her that was fine but maybe she could just try replacing one glass with water. A week later she walked in a told me that she had quit her diet cola habit and within two weeks she had lost ten pounds! The key of course is watching what we eat and moving more but always speak to your doctor first before making any radical changes to your diet. I will never forget the joy on her face when this simple change resulted in weight loss.

The Students Came Out of the Closet

Early on in my career we had been instructed never to leave the students unattended during the class, but I had a bathroom emergency that I had to address so I chose to go when all of the students were on the floor doing their ab workout. I got them started and explained that I would be very quick and to stay put and keep doing their exercises until I returned. Well much to my surprise I came back into the room to find my twenty students missing. I gasped and then heard giggling from all of the closets in the room and they all bounded out…They had certainly got me.

A Ride in Your Elevator?

During my chair workout which is typically filled with smiling but very quiet well-behaved students we were doing Kegels. I have a few men in the class so as I was telling the ladies to contract their pelvic floor, I instructed the ladies to lift up their 'elevators,' a sensation where we can actually feel the uterus lifting up. I smiled as I always do when giving this instruction and said, "the men are wondering what we are doing." To which a lady who was in my class for the first and last time, said, "yes and they are wondering if they can have a ride!" The entire class burst out laughing including me. Unfortunately, I never saw her again but we all appreciated the humour.

Have You Ever Done Step Before?

It was the start of a new September session and there were a few new faces in my class, so I went around introducing myself. Just when I thought I was done I noticed a lady on the far right who looked a bit out of place. I approached her and asked her if she had ever done Step before to which she replied emphatically, "yes." How interesting I thought to myself as her step was upside down with the risers resting on top. I flipped it over for her and told her that in my class we do it this way.

The Wrong Colour!

In the facility that I work for we have colour coded shoe tags that tell the staff what program the students have paid for. Because my classes can be so full I do this quite often to make certain that the students are in the right room. I could clearly see that a new lady in our midst had the wrong colour shoe tag for my class and I told her she needed to head to another room to find her proper spot. Well as it turns out she was a black woman who thought I was telling her that she could not be in my class because of the colour of her skin. She backed me up against the emergency door and put her nose right to mine, asking me if "I had a problem with her colour!" This upset me terribly as I have friends from all backgrounds. I could not believe how she was misunderstanding me. I tried not to laugh because she was clearly upset but I had to tell her that the colour of her shoe tag was wrong. Oh boy. She was mad, left and never came back.

I Have a Big Problem with You!

You never want to hear your boss say these words, but Shawna spoke them clearly into the phone, near the end of my first 12 weeks of teaching. I was freaking out and she knew it. My confidence was a bit low and she played upon it well. "I have a big problem with you Beth. The students love your classes so much that I am going to have to open another one back to back to accommodate the people on the waiting list!" I can still remember this conversation and how happy it made me to hear that all of my hard work learning how to teach fitness was paying off!

My Students Have the Best Butts!

I tell my students this all of the time because it is true. I spent quite a bit of time in the hospital vising my ailing father who was in there for one year awaiting a long-term care bed. During that time, I got to see many people in hospital gowns with absolutely flat buttocks. I am proud to say that my students have nicely proportioned buttocks. Well one of my students turned around in class recently and showed us that when she was in ballet school, they were taught to isolate each cheek. She was able to lift her left cheek without moving her right and before you know it, several of us were lined up in front of the mirrors seeing if we could do the same. We looked fairly silly I am certain, and we had a great laugh.

The Swearing Senior

I will never forget the student who attended my classes for one twelve-week session. She was close to 80 years old and very petite. She was a real sweetie but unfortunately whenever she missed a step in the choreography she would swear loudly. She was very close to me and each time I would hear her curse it would throw me off my game because it was so shocking to hear this tiny senior swear like a trucker! At first, I found it humorous but eventually I had to ask her to stop because she would make so many errors each class that it began to affect my mood.

Forgotten Shoes

It happens to the best of us. We forget one shoe or both. This is not so bad if you are a student but when you are the teacher and are facing three or four hours of aerobic classes, it can be a big problem. I do my best to pack my bag the night before but somehow I forgot my gym shoes. My 6:30am class wasn't bad as I simply called the exercises but there was not enough time to get to a store for my next three classes.

I decided that I was just going to have to muster through in my bare socks and as I came out of the locker room heading toward my next class, and angel student appeared with a large gift bag. It was close to my birthday and she had picked up two pair of fitness shoes for me to try. I was speechless as she expressed regret that they were not gift wrapped! I could not believe my luck. It was such an amazing coincidence. What a great gift in so many ways.

Making An Entrance

It was the first day of the fall session in September. The class was packed with approximately fifty students. All eyes were on me as I walked to the front of the room to introduce myself. I placed my water bottle down on a ledge near my spot and turned to address the crowd when all of a sudden I heard a loud crash and commotion erupted to my right. The floor was now covered in shards of glass. For some reason the wall clock had been propped up on the shelf beside my water bottle and I had caused it to fall unknowingly. Instead of welcoming everybody in, I now had to ask everyone to leave so that the janitor could sweep the floor in its entirety. "Welcome back everyone. Now could you please leave?" We laughed but I was terribly embarrassed.

Fireman Visits

On at least two occasions in my twenty-year career, we had emergency visits to the gym by firemen. Thankfully our class went on uninterrupted, but the firemen did come into the room to check the on the fire extinguishers. This would bring elicit quite a reaction from my primarily female class, who were between 65 and 78 years old. One student in particular loved to talk to them directly, saying that she was feeling uneasy and needed CPR. The rest of the class would giggle and from that point on she would threaten to pull the fire alarm regularly just to spice up the class!

Take It Off

If there is one thing that I have learned from my years in the business, seniors speak their minds often because they want to be heard and they want action. Well early on in my career, I was leading an aerobics class and I became quite hot. I kept teaching but removed my sweatshirt in the process, as I had an exercise top underneath. One of the gentleman in the back called out, "take it all off!" I was so shocked that I lost my place and began laughing out loud. This man loved to make me laugh and it worked often.

Monkey See, Monkey Do

I taught water aerobics or aquafit for four years when I first began teaching. I never got in the water with my participants because I had to run to the fitness room for my next class as soon as ours ended. I therefore had to act like I was in the water when moving on the deck and this can be quite humorous to anyone watching as it becomes quite the balance challenge for the instructor. One fond memory I have is whenever I was stretching the clients at the end of the workout, I would have them performing a stretch and if I began to lose my balance while on one leg, I would hop. Suddenly the entire class would start hopping along with me. Makes me grin to think back on those moments. Monkey see, monkey do. This also happens with new students in aerobics. When I give verbal cues, I often signal with my hands as well. Occasionally I will have one or two students mimicking the hand movements along with me and I suggest that they are actually after my job!

Running Late

I live quite far from my primary place of work. It can take forty-five minutes on a good day and if you add in snow or freezing rain, it can take two hours. There was a snowstorm and I found myself running into the building ten minutes after the scheduled start time. As I tore down the hallway, peeling off my jacket and scarf, I could hear my Step students, stepping without me but I could not hear any music. I was upset thinking that my class has been given to another teacher, which would mean no pay for the hour but as I grew closer and walked into the room, I saw one of my students in my place, grinning from ear to ear, calling as best he could the moves that we all knew so well. The class erupted in applause, not just for me but for Mark who made my job look too easy! Thanks Mark.

Ghostly Grab

I often use a church hall for my classes and on two separate occasions when we were using the basement room for yoga, I felt someone grab me from behind. Both times I giggled and look behind me thinking that my students were playing a trick on me, but I would find them deeply focused on their pose and nowhere near me that would allow them to easily reach out and commit the act. It happened during Chair Pose where the body lowers down into an easy squat with the hands reaching up in the air. Someone or something gently cupped my buttocks in two different classes, weeks apart. The second time I turned around and exclaimed "stop it," and saw blank stares looking my way. I think there is a good humoured ghost living in that basement and I will never forget that haunting experience.

Managing Injuries

I have had my share of injuries and because I don't want to be the focus of attention, I downplay any situation so that I can get my job done. While packing for my busy day ahead, I decided to jam everything into one large, newly acquired gym bag, instead of carrying three smaller bags. I threw the bag up and over my shoulder but realized that I had left my water bottle down on the ground. Instead of squatting down, I bent forward and my bag swung around to the front of my body, putting excessive pressure on my lower back. I felt a pain immediately but figured it would be fine in time. Turns out I had slipped a disc but did not know it yet. I managed to get through my day by simply calling the moves but in my home class that night, I found myself unable to get up off of the floor after leading the class through the stretching segment. I just laughed saying that the exercises were so hard I could not walk. I had done myself in. Everyone giggled and were none the wiser. I will never forget that pain.

Rental Woes

I have rented many locations over the years and I have had my share of troubles with rooms being unusable because of power outages, locked doors and failing heating or air conditioning systems. One cold day in February my early morning Saturday class was set to take place in an old park building. When I arrived, the door was completely frozen shut by an ice storm that had rolled through during the night. No matter how hard I tried I could not get the key in the door. The students arrived and I said I have to cancel class because I could not get in. Well two of the male students went around to the back of the building to see if they could get in the back door while another drove home and got some magic liquid to spray in the mechanism. I was quite happy to cancel class and go have breakfast but they would not give up until we were all inside. We started a bit late but the show went on successfully. Thanks Steve.

Fired For Making Muscles

I am a personal trainer and part of my job is to make my clients stronger. I have always wanted to have a defined body, but I learned the hard way that some women do not want to have muscles. Lady X hired me to help her lose weight, so I put her on a training program that included daily muscle conditioning exercises and various forms of cardio. After two weeks she was looking wonderful but when I arrived for our session she was very upset. She looked down at her leg and pointed to a bulge in her thigh. "What is that?" she asked. I explained that it was her quadriceps muscle and that it was likely a result of the squats that she had been doing. She said she didn't want muscles and cancelled our contract. I still shake my head in disbelief, but I now make certain to explain to all of my clients that we just might make some muscles while working together.

Watch Your Keys

Some students like to keep their personal items near my things at the front of the class. I am not sure why but perhaps they feel that they can have their eyes on their belongings and on me at the same time. Well Susan and I were both driving Jetta's at the time and even though she had not driven to class that day, she put her purse down next to mine. After everyone had gone and I had packed up the equipment, I reached for my car keys and could not find them anywhere. I emptied all of my bags three times and my pockets too and then realized that Susan must have picked up my keys out of habit, thinking they were hers. Here I was with no ability to drive away, no phone number for her cell and no idea where her family had gone to breakfast (they often left class and went directly to a restaurant). Thankfully I managed to find the cell number of her best friend and when I found Susan, we laughed about what she had done. I now keep my keys on a chain, hooked directly to my gym bag. Oh Susan, I do love you.

Energy Drink Madness

I used to teach a 6:45 am class and I would have to rise at 4:30 am in order to get ready and get there on time. Well as parent with three young kids and three jobs, occasionally fatigue took a hold. One of my students happened to have an energy drink in his bag (I won't say the name but it has the color red in the title) and he offered it to me thinking it might help to get me through my shift of classes. I drank half of it and I can tell you honestly that I had so much energy it frightened me off of ever drinking it again! I probably taught the best class of my career but it sure wasn't all me that day. Wow, what a crazy experience. I can see why they are so popular but encourage everyone to avoid these drinks and just get plenty of rest and eat well.

Beth's Favorite Motivational Self-Help Books

Bailey, Chris. *The Productivity Project-Accomplishing More by Managing Your Time, Attention and Energy.* Toronto: Random House Canada, 2016.

Ban Breathmach, Sarah. *The Simple Abundance Journal of Gratitude.* New York: Warner Books, Inc., 1996.

Byrne, Rhonda. *The Power.* New York: Atria Books, 2010.

Byrne, Rhonda. *The Magic.* New York: Atria Books, 2012.

Chodron, Pema. *The Places That Scare You*. Boston, Massachusetts: Shambhala Publications, 2001.

Chodron, Pema. *When Things Fall Apart.* Boston, Massachusetts: Shambhala Publications, 1997.

Daniluk, Julie. *Slimming Meals That Heal.* Toronto: Random House Canada, 2014.

Esmonde-White, Miranda. *Aging Backwards. 10 Years Younger and 10 Years Lighter in 30 Minutes a Day.* Toronto: Random House Canada, 2014.

Grierson, Bruce. *What Makes Olga Run? The Mystery of the 90-Something Track Star, and What She Can Teach Us About Living Longer, Happier Lives.* Toronto: Random House Canada, 2014.

Kondo, Marie. *The Life-changing Magic of Tidying Up: The Japanese Art of Decluttering and Organizing.* New York: Ten Speed, 2014.

Singer, Michael A. *The Untethered Soul: The Journey Beyond Yourself.* Oakland, CA: New Harbinger Publications, 2007.

Tolle, Eckhart. *The Power of Now: A Guide to Spiritual Enlightenment.* Vancouver, BC: Namaste Publishing, 1997.

Wolynn, Mark. *It Didn't Start With You. How Inherited Family Trauma Shapes Who We Are and How to End The Cycle.* New York: Viking, 2016.

Credits and Acknowledgments

All photographs by Gnarly Tree Photography. Thank you Allan for your professionalism and patience.

Male Model: Peter Vatne

I would like to thank my husband Peter for taking the time to sit and pose for some of the photographs and for all of his input into making my dream a reality.

I also need to thank my good friend, Christiane Poirier, for translating some of the student testimonials from French to English.

ABOUT THE AUTHOR

Beth Oldfield

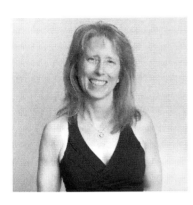 Beth Oldfield has been teaching fitness for 20 years in Pointe-Claire, Quebec. With a Bachelor of Arts and a Diploma in Education from McGill University, she is a Fitness Instructor Specialist and a Personal Training Specialist as well as an Older Adult Specialist with Canfitpro.

Participants ranging in age from 20 to 85 years young embrace her enthusiasm and energy by filling her classes to capacity. Beth's mission is to educate and motivate her students to be the best that they can be in body, mind and spirit. Her specialities include Aerobics/Step/Muscle Conditioning/Yoga/Line Dance and Essentrics.

Beth currently commutes from the country where she has been living for 25 years with her husband Peter. Together they have designed and built two homes with their own hands and raised three beautiful children who are now successful adults. When she is not teaching, reading or writing short stories and updating her weekly fitness blog at betholdfield.ca, she is cooking delicious gluten free food.

Connect with Beth at www.betholdfield.ca.

Printed in Great Britain
by Amazon